MRI Basic Principles and Applications

MRI Basic Principles and Applications

Brian M. Dale, PhD MBA

Mark A. Brown, PhD

Richard C. Semelka, MD

FIFTH EDITION

WILEY Blackwell

This edition first published 2015 © 2015 by John Wiley & Sons, Ltd

Registered office: John Wiley & Sons, Ltd, The Atrium, Southern Gate, Chichester, West Sussex, PO19 8SQ, UK

Editorial offices: 9600 Garsington Road, Oxford, OX4 2DQ, UK
　　　　　　　111 River Street, Hoboken, NJ 07030-5774, USA

For details of our global editorial offices, for customer services and for information about how to apply for permission to reuse the copyright material in this book please see our website at www.wiley.com/wiley-blackwell

Library of Congress Cataloging-in-Publication Data

Dale, Brian M., author.
  MRI : basic principles and applications / Brian M. Dale, Mark A. Brown, and Richard C. Semelka. – Fifth edition.
　　　　　p. ; cm.
  Preceded by MRI / Mark A. Brown, Richard C. Semelka. 4th ed. c2010.
  Includes bibliographical references and index.
  ISBN 978-1-119-01305-1 (pbk.)
  I. Brown, Mark A., 1955- , author. II. Semelka, Richard C., author. III. Brown, Mark A., 1955- MRI. Preceded by (work): IV. Title.
  [DNLM: 1. Magnetic Resonance Imaging–methods. WN 185]
  RC78.7.N83
  616.07′548–dc23
　　　　　　　　　　　　　　　　　　　　　　　　　　　　　　　　　2015015322

A catalogue record for this book is available from the British Library.

Wiley also publishes its books in a variety of electronic formats. Some content that appears in print may not be available in electronic books.

Set in 9.5/13pt, MeridienLTStd by SPi Global, Chennai, India.

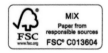

Contents

Preface

Magnetic Resonance Imaging (MRI) continues to be an integral component of medical imaging. New measurement techniques and applications continue to be developed nearly thirty years after the initial clinical scanners were installed. Even so, the basic principles behind the measurement techniques remain as true today as then. This book was written to present the fundamental concepts of MRI in a clear and concise manner, minimizing the mathematical formalism yet providing a foundation to understand the results that are obtained with today's clinical scanners.

Since the fourth edition, parallel imaging and high channel-count coil arrays have become mainstream clinical tools. We have added material describing the physics behind these modern techniques. We have also added a focus on material that is relevant to radiologist board exams. Such material is highlighted in the text and will now be easier to find and identify. It is interspersed with other material that remains important for a deeper understanding of the physics of MRI and provides additional clarity. New and updated figures are included throughout the book.

As always, many people must be thanked for their help in this. First, we would like to thank the technical staff at the Siemens Training and Development Center and the faculty, fellows, and staff at the University of North Carolina for their interest in this project and their assistance in its completion. In addition, thanks to Wolfgang Rehwald, James R. MacFall, and H. Cecil Charles for providing images. Finally, thanks to our families for their support and patience in this project.

B.M. Dale
M.A. Brown
R.C. Semelka

ABR study guide topics

Where you see text within lines and accompanied by the logo, this indicates content that would be especially useful for those studying for the American Boards of Radiology.

The list below indicates the location of that content throughout the book.

Magnetic fields
   Magnetic susceptibility – 1.6
   Types of magnetic materials – 1.6
   Magnetic Fields (B) – 1.1
   Magnetic moment interaction with an external field (B0): the Larmor equation and precessional frequency – 1.4
   Net magnetization due to B0 and field strength – 1.5
Nuclear MR and excitation – 2.1
MR signal properties
   Spin density (proton) – 3.1
   T2 (transverse) relaxation – 3.2
   *T2** relaxation – 3.2
   T1 (longitudinal) relaxation – 3.1
   T1 weighting, *T2* weighting, proton density-weighting – 6.1
Pulse sequences and contrast mechanisms
   Echo time (TE), repetition time (TR), and inversion time (TI) – 6.1, 6.4
   Spin-echo (SE) pulse sequences – 6.1
   Inversion-recovery spin-echo pulse sequences – 6.4
   Gradient-echo (GE or GRE) pulse sequences – 6.2
   Echo-planar (EPI) pulse sequences – 6.3
   Fast- or turbo-spin-echo (FSE) pulse sequences – 6.1
   Manipulation of pulse sequence characteristics – 7.1
MR instrumentation
   Static magnetic field (B0) systems – 14.2
   Gradient fields and the gradient subsystem – 14.3
   Shimming and shim coils – 14.2
   Radiofrequency transmitter (B1) subsystem – 14.4
   Radiofrequency receiver subsystem – 14.5
   Radiofrequency coils – 14.5

Spatial localization
    Slice-selection – 4.2
    Phase-encoding – 4.4
    Frequency-encoding – 4.3
Two-dimensional Fourier transform (2DFT) image reconstruction – 5.3
    k-space description – 5.5
    Methods of filling k-space – 5.6, 5.7
Image characteristics
    Factors affecting spatial resolution – 4.2, 4.3, 4.4
    Factors affecting signal-to-noise ratio (SNR) – 5.4, 7.3.2
    Tradeoffs among spatial resolution, SNR, and acquisition time – 5.4, 7.3
    Factors affecting image contrast – 7.1, 7.3.1
Contrast agents – 15
Spatial saturation and fat suppression – 8.1, 8.3, 8.4
Special acquisition techniques
    Angiography – 11
    Diffusion, perfusion and neuro imaging – 12.1, 12.2, 17.3.1
    Functional MRI (fMRI) – 12.3
    Magnetization transfer contrast (MTC) – 8.2
Artifacts – 9
Safety, bioeffects, and FDA limits
    Static magnetic field (ferromagnetic materials) – 16.1
    Radiofrequency field (heating) – 16.4
    Gradient field (nerve stimulation) – 16.3
    Contrast agent safety issues – 16.5

CHAPTER 1

Production of net magnetization

Magnetic resonance (MR) is a measurement technique used to examine atoms and molecules. It is based upon the interaction between an applied magnetic field and a particle that possesses spin and charge. While electrons and other subatomic particles possess spin (or more precisely, spin angular momentum) and can be examined using MR techniques, this book focuses on nuclei and the use of MR techniques for their study, formally known as Nuclear Magnetic Resonance, or NMR. Nuclear spin, or more precisely nuclear spin angular momentum, is one of several intrinsic properties of an atom and its value depends on the precise atomic composition. Every element in the Periodic Table except argon and cerium has at least one naturally occurring isotope that possesses nuclear spin. Thus, in principle, nearly every element can be examined using MR, and the basic ideas of resonance absorption and relaxation are common for all of these elements. The precise details will vary from nucleus to nucleus and from system to system.

1.1 Magnetic fields

 Magnetic fields are produced by and surround electric currents, whether these currents are macroscopic currents such as those running through wires or microscopic currents such as those around an atom of iron. The magnetic field can be represented as a vector, meaning that it has both a magnitude and a direction, and is usually denoted by the variable B.[1] For example, the B field at the center of a circular loop of current-carrying wire points in the direction of the axis of the loop (perpendicular to the plane of the loop and therefore perpendicular to the current flow) and it has a magnitude that is proportional to the current in the loop. The magnitude of the field is related to the strength of the magnetic force on wires or magnetic materials, and the direction of the field is perpendicular to the direction of the force.

---

[1] In this book, vector quantities with direction and magnitude are indicated by boldface type while scalar quantities that are magnitude only are indicated by regular typeface.

MRI Basic Principles and Applications, Fifth Edition.
Brian M. Dale, Mark A. Brown and Richard C. Semelka.
© 2015 John Wiley & Sons, Ltd. Published 2015 by John Wiley & Sons, Ltd.

Magnetic fields often vary over time and/or space, and will be coupled to the electric field, producing electromagnetic waves. Magnetic fields, particularly those in electromagnetic waves, are characterized by their frequency (the time between two consecutive "peaks" in the field). In MR, there are magnetic fields, which are constant in time, which vary at acoustic frequencies (a few kilohertz), and which vary at radio frequencies (RF) (several megahertz).

1.2 Nuclear spin

The structure of an atom is an essential component of the MR experiment. Atoms consist of three fundamental particles: protons, which possess a positive charge; neutrons, which have no charge; and electrons, which have a negative charge. The protons and neutrons are located in the nucleus or core of an atom; thus all nuclei are positively charged. The electrons are located in shells or orbitals surrounding the nucleus. The characteristic chemical reactions of elements depend upon the particular number of each of these particles. The properties most commonly used to categorize elements are the atomic number and the atomic weight. The atomic number is the number of protons in the nucleus and is the primary index used to differentiate atoms. All atoms of an element have the same atomic number and undergo the same chemical reactions. The atomic weight is the sum of the number of protons and the number of neutrons. Atoms with the same atomic number but different atomic weights are called isotopes. Isotopes of an element will undergo the same chemical reactions, but at different reaction rates.

A third property of the nucleus is spin or intrinsic spin angular momentum. Classically, nuclei with spin can be considered to be always rotating about an axis at a constant rate. This self-rotation axis is perpendicular to the direction of rotation (Figure 1.1). A limited number of values for the spin are found in nature; that is, the spin, I, is quantized to certain discrete values. These values depend on the atomic number and atomic weight of the particular nucleus. There are three groups of values for I: zero, integral, and half-integral values. A nucleus has no spin ($I = 0$) if it has an even atomic weight and an even atomic number; for example, ^{12}C (6 protons and 6 neutrons) or ^{16}O (8 protons and 8 neutrons). Such a nucleus does not interact with an external magnetic field and cannot be studied using MR. A nucleus has an integral value for I (e.g., 1, 2, 3) if it has an even atomic weight and an odd atomic number; for example, ^{2}H (1 proton and 1 neutron) or ^{6}Li (3 protons and 3 neutrons). A nucleus has a half-integral value for I (e.g., 1/2, 3/2, 5/2) if it has an odd atomic weight. Table 1.1 lists the spin and isotopic composition for several elements commonly found in biological systems. The ^{1}H nucleus, consisting of a single proton, is a natural choice for probing the body using MR techniques for several reasons. It has a spin of 1/2 and is the most

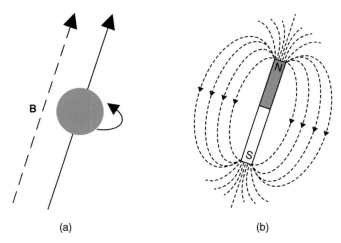

(a)   (b)

Figure 1.1 A rotating nucleus (spin) with a positive charge produces a magnetic field known as the magnetic moment oriented parallel to the axis of rotation (a). This arrangement is analogous to a bar magnet in which the magnetic field is considered to be oriented from the south to the north pole (b).

Table 1.1   Constants for Selected Nuclei of Biological Interest.

Element	Nuclear composition		Nuclear spin I	Gyromagnetic ratio γ (MHz T⁻¹)	% Natural abundance	ω at 1.5 T (MHz)
	Protons	Neutrons				
¹H, protium	1	0	1/2	42.5774	99.985	63.8646
²H, deuterium	1	1	1	6.53896	0.015	9.8036
³He	2	1	1/2	32.436	0.000138	48.6540
⁶Li	3	3	1	6.26613	7.5	9.39919
⁷Li	3	4	3/2	16.5483	92.5	24.8224
¹²C	6	6	0	0	98.90	0
¹³C	6	7	1/2	10.7084	1.10	16.0621
¹⁴N	7	7	1	3.07770	99.634	4.6164
¹⁵N	7	8	1/2	4.3173	0.366	6.4759
¹⁶O	8	8	0	0	99.762	0
¹⁷O	8	9	5/2	5.7743	0.038	8.6614
¹⁹F	9	10	1/2	40.0776	100	60.1164
²³Na	11	12	3/2	11.2686	100	16.9029
³¹P	15	16	1/2	17.2514	100	25.8771
¹²⁹Xe	54	75	1/2	11.8604	26.4	17.7906

Source: Adapted from Ian Mills (ed.), *Quantities, Units, and Symbols in Physical Chemistry*, IUPAC, Physical Chemistry Division, Blackwell, Oxford, UK, 1989.

abundant isotope for hydrogen. Its response to an applied magnetic field is one of the largest found in nature. Since the body is composed of tissues that contain primarily water and fat, both of which contain hydrogen, a significant MR signal can be produced naturally by normal tissues.

While a rigorous mathematical description of a nucleus with spin and its interactions requires the use of quantum mechanical principles, most of MR can be described using the concepts of classical mechanics, particularly in describing the actions of a nucleus with spin. The subsequent discussions of MR phenomena in this book use a classical approach. In addition, while the concepts of resonance absorption and relaxation apply to all nuclei with spin, the descriptions in this book focus on ^{1}H (commonly referred to as a proton) since most imaging experiments visualize the ^{1}H nucleus.

1.3 Nuclear magnetic moments

Recall that the nucleus is the location of the positively charged protons. When this charge rotates due to the nuclear spin, a local magnetic field or magnetic moment is induced about the nucleus. This magnetic moment will be oriented parallel to the axis of rotation. Since the nuclear spin is constant in magnitude, its associated magnetic moment will also be constant in magnitude. This magnetic moment is fundamental to MR. A bar magnet provides a useful analogy. A bar magnet has a north and a south pole, or, more precisely, a magnitude and orientation to the magnetic field can be defined. The axis of rotation for a nucleus with spin can similarly be viewed as a vector with a definite orientation and magnitude (Figure 1.1). This orientation of the nuclear spin and the changes induced in it due to the experimental manipulations that the nucleus undergoes provide the basis for the MR signal.

In general, MR measurements are made on collections of spins rather than on an individual spin. It is convenient to consider such a collection both as individual spins acting independently (a "microscopic" picture) and as a single entity (a "macroscopic" picture). For many concepts, the two pictures provide equivalent results, even though the microscopic picture is more complete. Conversion between the two pictures requires the principles of statistical mechanics. While necessary for a complete understanding of MR phenomena, the nature of this conversion is beyond the scope of this book. However, the macroscopic picture is sufficient for an adequate description for most concepts presented in this book. When necessary, the microscopic picture will be used.

1.4 Larmor precession

Consider an arbitrary volume of tissue containing hydrogen atoms (protons) in the absence of an external magnetic field. Each proton has a spin vector (or magnetic moment) of equal magnitude. However, the spin vectors for the entire collection of protons within the tissue are randomly oriented in all directions; there is a continuous distribution of the spin orientations. Performing a vector addition (head-to-toe) of these spin vectors produces a zero sum; that is, no net magnetization is observed in the tissue (Figure 1.2).

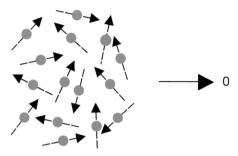

Figure 1.2 Microscopic and macroscopic pictures of a collection of spins in the absence of an external magnetic field. In the absence of a magnetic field, the spins have their axes oriented randomly (microscopic picture, left side of figure). The vector sum of these spin vectors is zero (macroscopic picture, right side).

If the tissue is placed inside a magnetic field B_0, the individual protons begin to rotate perpendicular to, or precess about, the magnetic field. The spin vectors for the protons are tilted slightly away from the axis of the magnetic field, but each axis of precession is parallel to B_0. This precession is at a constant rate and occurs because of the interaction of the magnetic field with the spinning positive charge of the nucleus. By convention, B_0 and the axis of precession are defined to be oriented in the z direction of a Cartesian coordinate system. (This convention is not universally followed, but it is the prevailing convention.) The motion of each proton can be described by a set of coordinates perpendicular (x and y) and parallel (z) to B_0. In the absence of other interactions the perpendicular, or transverse, coordinates are nonzero but vary cyclically with time as the proton precesses, while the parallel or longitudinal coordinate is constant with time (Figure 1.3). The rate or frequency

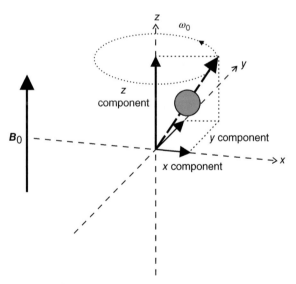

Figure 1.3 Inside a magnetic field, a proton precesses or revolves about the magnetic field. The precessional axis is parallel to the main magnetic field, B_0. The z component of the spin vector (projection of the spin onto the z axis) is the component of interest because it does not change in magnitude or direction as the proton precesses. The x and y components vary with time at a frequency ω_0 proportional to B_0 as expressed by equation (1.1).

of precession is proportional to the strength of the magnetic field and is expressed by the following equation, known as the Larmor equation:

$$\omega_0 = \gamma B_0 \tag{1.1}$$

where ω_0 is the Larmor frequency in megahertz (MHz),[2] B_0 is the magnetic field strength in tesla (T) that the proton experiences, and γ is a constant for each nucleus in MHz/T, known as the gyromagnetic ratio. Values for γ and ω at 1.5 T for several nuclei are tabulated in Table 1.1.

An alternate picture known as a rotating frame of reference or rotating coordinate system is often used in MR. It is a convenient view when describing objects that undergo rotational motion. When viewed using in a rotating frame of reference, the coordinate system rotates about one axis while the other two axes vary with time. By choosing a suitable axis and rate of rotation for the coordinate system, the rotating object appears stationary.

For MR experiments, a convenient rotating frame uses the z axis, parallel to B_0, as the axis of rotation while the x and y axes rotate at the Larmor frequency, ω_0. When viewed in this fashion, the precessing spin appears stationary in space with a fixed set of x, y, and z coordinates. Regardless of whether a stationary or rotating coordinate system is used, M_0 is of fixed amplitude and is parallel to the main magnetic field. For all subsequent discussions in this book, a rotating frame of reference with the rotation axis parallel to B_0 is used when describing the motion of the protons.

1.5 Net magnetization

If a vector addition is performed, as before, for the spin vectors inside the magnetic field, the results will be slightly different than for the sum outside the field. In the direction perpendicular to B_0, despite the precession of each spin, the spin orientations are still randomly distributed (covering a complete range of x and y values, both positive and negative) just as they were outside the magnetic field. There is therefore still no net magnetization perpendicular to B_0. However, in the direction parallel to B_0, there is a different result. Because there is an orientation to the precessional axis of the proton that is constant with time, there is a constant, nonzero interaction or coupling between the proton and B_0, known

---

[2]In many physics discussions, ω (Greek letter omega) is used to represent angular frequency, with units of s^{-1}, while cyclical frequency, in units of Hertz (Hz), is represented either by ν (Greek letter nu) or f. A factor of 2π (explicitly in the equation or hidden in the constant) is necessary to convert from angular to cyclical frequency. In imaging derivations, the Larmor equation is usually expressed as equation 1.1, using ω with units of Hz to represent cyclical frequency. To minimize confusion, we follow the imaging tradition throughout this book.

as the Zeeman interaction. Instead of a continuous range of values, this coupling causes the z component to be quantized to a limited or discrete number of values. For the ^{1}H nucleus, there are only two possible values for the z component: parallel or along $\boldsymbol{B}_0$ and antiparallel or against $\boldsymbol{B}_0$. This coupling also causes a difference in energy ΔE between these two orientations that is proportional to B_0 (Figure 1.4). This leads to a slight excess of positive z values compared to negative z values as described in detail below. If a vector sum is performed on this collection of protons, the x and y components sum to zero but a nonzero, positive z component will be left, the net magnetization $\boldsymbol{M}_0$. In addition, since the z axis is the axis of rotation, $\boldsymbol{M}_0$ does not vary with time.

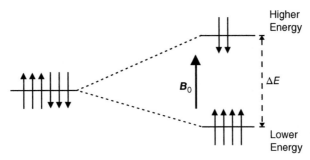

Figure 1.4 Zeeman diagram. In the absence of a magnetic field (left side of figure), a collection of spins will have the configurations of z components equal in energy so that there is no preferential alignment between the spin-up and spin-down orientations. In the presence of a magnetic field (right side), the spin-up orientation (parallel to $\boldsymbol{B}_0$) is of lower energy and its configuration contains more spins than does the higher-energy spin-down configuration. The difference in energy ΔE between the two levels is proportional to $\boldsymbol{B}_0$.

The result of the Zeeman interaction is that spins in the two orientations, parallel (also known as spin up) and antiparallel (spin down), have different energies. Those spins oriented parallel to $\boldsymbol{B}_0$ are of lower energy than those oriented antiparallel. For a collection of protons, more will be oriented parallel to $\boldsymbol{B}_0$ than antiparallel; that is, there is residual polarization of the spins induced parallel to the magnetic field (Figure 1.5a). The exact number of protons in each energy level can be predicted by a distribution function known as the Boltzmann distribution:

$$N_{\text{UPPER}}/N_{\text{LOWER}} = e^{-\Delta E/kT} \tag{1.2}$$

where k is Boltzmann's constant, 1.381×10^{-23} J K^{-1} and N_{UPPER} and N_{LOWER} are the number of protons in the upper and lower energy levels, respectively. Since the separation between the energy levels ΔE depends on the field strength B_0, the exact number of spins in each level also depends on B_0 and the difference increases with increasing B_0. For a collection of protons at body temperature (310 K) at 1.5 T, there will typically be an excess of ~1:10^6 protons in the lower level out of the approximately 10^{25} protons within the tissue. This unequal number of protons in each energy level means that the vector sum of spins will be nonzero and will point along the magnetic field. In other words, the tissue will become polarized or magnetized in the presence of $\boldsymbol{B}_0$ with a value $\boldsymbol{M}_0$, known as the net magnetization. The orientation of this net magnetization will be in the same direction as $\boldsymbol{B}_0$ and, in the absence of other interactions, will be constant with respect to time (Figure 1.5b).

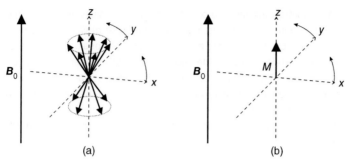

Figure 1.5 Microscopic (a) and macroscopic (b) pictures of a collection of spins in the presence of an external magnetic field. Each spin precesses about the magnetic field. If a rotating frame of reference is used with a rotation rate of ω_0, the collection of protons appears stationary. Whereas the z components are one of two values (one positive and one negative), the x and y components can be any value, positive or negative. The spins will appear to track along two cones, one with a positive z component and one with a negative z component. Because there are more spins in the upper cone, there will be a nonzero vector sum $\boldsymbol{M}_0$, the net magnetization. It will be of constant magnitude and parallel to $\boldsymbol{B}_0$.

1.6 Susceptibility and magnetic materials

 For most materials (including biological tissues), the magnitude and direction of $\boldsymbol{M}_0$ is proportional to $\boldsymbol{B}_0$:

$$M_0 = \chi B_0 \tag{1.3}$$

where χ is known as the bulk magnetic susceptibility or simply the magnetic susceptibility. This arrangement with $\boldsymbol{M}_0$ aligned along the magnetic field with no transverse component is the normal, or equilibrium, configuration for the protons. This configuration of spins has the lowest energy and is the arrangement to which the protons will naturally try to return following any perturbations such as energy absorption. This induced magnetization, $\boldsymbol{M}_0$, is the source of signal for all of the MR experiments. Consequently, all other things being equal, the greater the field strength, the greater the value of $\boldsymbol{M}_0$ and the greater the potential MR signal.

The magnetic susceptibility describes the response of a substance to the applied magnetic field. While a complete analysis of the origin of this response is beyond the scope of this book, it is useful to describe the three levels of response that are encountered in MR. A diamagnetic response is found in all materials, arising from the electrons surrounding the nuclei. It is a very weak response (χ is very small and negative) except for superconductors. The diamagnetic response produces a slight repulsive force and is the only response for most materials, including tissue. A paramagnetic response is larger in magnitude than a diamagnetic response, but still relatively weak (χ is small but positive). It is found in molecules where there are so-called unpaired electrons, which align themselves in response to the external field and produce a mild attractive force. The final response level is known as ferromagnetic, typically found in certain metals in which χ is very large and positive. The atoms in ferromagnetic materials align with each other to form relatively large (still microscopic) magnetic domains. The alignment of these domains produces a strong attractive force in response to an external field and also leaves the ferromagnetic material with a permanent residual magnetization after the external field is removed. While diamagnetic and paramagnetic materials are safe to be in or near MR scanners, ferromagnetic materials should remain outside the scan room.

CHAPTER 2

Concepts of magnetic resonance

In its most basic form, the MR experiment can be analyzed in terms of energy transfer. During the measurement process, the patient or sample is exposed to energy at the correct frequency that will be absorbed. A short time later, this energy is reemitted, at which time it can be detected and processed. A detailed presentation of the processes involved in this absorption and reemission requires the use of linear response theory, which is beyond the scope of this book. However, a general description of the nature of the molecular interactions is useful. In particular, the relationship between the molecular picture and the macroscopic picture provides an avenue for explanation of the principles of MR.

2.1 Radiofrequency excitation

Chapter 1 described the formation of the net magnetization, M_0, by the protons within a sample. The entire field of MR is based on the manipulation of M_0. The simplest manipulation involves the application of a short burst, or pulse, of radiofrequency (RF) energy. This pulse, referred to as an excitation pulse, typically contains a narrow range or bandwidth of frequencies centered around a central frequency. During the pulse, the protons absorb a portion of this energy at a particular frequency. The particular frequency absorbed is proportional to the magnetic field B_0; the equation relating the two is the Larmor equation, equation (1.1). Following the pulse, the protons reemit the energy at the same frequency.

The frequency of energy absorbed by an individual proton is defined very precisely by the magnetic field that the proton experiences due to the quantized nature of the spin orientation. When a proton is irradiated with energy of the correct frequency (ω_0), it is excited from the lower energy (spin up) orientation to the higher energy (spin down) orientation (Figure 2.1). At the same time, a proton in the higher energy level is stimulated to release its energy and will go to the lower energy level. The energy difference (ΔE) between the two levels is exactly proportional to the frequency ω_0 and thus the magnetic field B_0:

$$\Delta E = h\omega_0 = h\gamma B_0 \tag{2.1}$$

MRI Basic Principles and Applications, Fifth Edition.
Brian M. Dale, Mark A. Brown and Richard C. Semelka.
© 2015 John Wiley & Sons, Ltd. Published 2015 by John Wiley & Sons, Ltd.

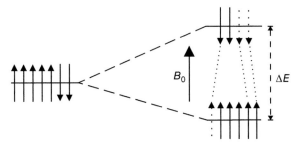

Figure 2.1 Energy absorption (microscopic). The difference in energy ΔE between the two configurations (spin up and spin down) is proportional to the magnetic field strength B_0 and the corresponding precessional frequency ω_0, as expressed in Equation (2.1). When energy at this frequency is applied, a spin from the lower-energy state is excited to the upper-energy state. Also, a spin from the upper-energy state is stimulated to give up its energy and relax to the lower-energy state. Because there are more spins in the lower-energy state, there is a net absorption of energy by the spins in the sample.

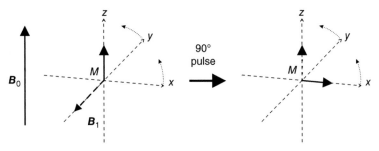

Figure 2.2 Energy absorption (macroscopic). In a rotating frame of reference, the RF pulse broadcast at the resonant frequency ω_0 can be treated as an additional magnetic field B_1 oriented perpendicular to B_0. When energy is applied at the appropriate frequency, the spins absorb it and M rotates into the transverse plane. The initial direction of rotation is perpendicular to both B_0 and B_1. The amount of resulting rotation of M is known as the pulse flip angle.

where h is Planck's constant, 6.626×10^{-34} Js. Only energy at this frequency stimulates transitions between the spin up and spin down energy levels. This quantized energy absorption is known as resonance absorption and the associated frequency is known as the resonant frequency.

Although an individual proton absorbs the radiofrequency energy, it is more useful to discuss the resonance condition by examining the effect of the energy absorption on M_0. For a large collection of protons such as in a volume of tissue, there is a significant amount of both absorption and emission occurring during the RF pulse. However, because there are more protons in the lower energy level (Figure 2.1), there will be a net absorption of energy by the tissue. The energy is applied as an RF pulse with a central frequency ω_{TR} and an orientation perpendicular to B_0, as indicated by an effective field B_1 (Figure 2.2). This orientation difference allows a coupling between the RF pulse and M_0 so that energy can be transferred to the protons. When the transmitter frequency matches the resonant frequency ($\omega_0 = \omega_{TR}$), the RF energy will be absorbed, which causes M_0 to rotate away from its equilibrium orientation.

The initial direction of rotation of M_0 is perpendicular to both B_0 and B_1. If the transmitter is left on long enough and at a high enough amplitude, the absorbed energy causes M_0 to rotate entirely into the transverse plane, a result known as a 90° pulse. When viewed in the rotating frame, the motion of M_0 is a simple vector rotation; however, the end result is the same whether a rotating or stationary frame of reference is used.

2.2 Radiofrequency signal detection

When the transmitter is turned off, the protons immediately begin to realign themselves and return to their original equilibrium orientation. They emit energy at frequency ω_0 as they do so. In addition, the net magnetization will begin to precess about B_0 similar to the behavior of a gyroscope when tilted away from a vertical axis. If a loop of wire (receiver) is placed perpendicular to the transverse plane, M_0 will induce a voltage in the wire during its precession. This induced voltage, the MR signal, is known as the FID, or free induction decay (Figure 2.3a). The initial magnitude of the FID signal depends on the value of M_0 immediately prior to the 90° pulse. The FID decays with time as more of the protons give up their absorbed energy through a process known as relaxation (see Chapter 3) and the coherence or uniformity of the proton motion is lost.

In general, three components of an MR signal are of interest: its magnitude or peak amplitude, its frequency, and its phase or direction relative to the RF transmitter phase (Figure 2.4). As mentioned previously, the signal magnitude is related to the value of M_0 immediately prior to the RF pulse. The signal frequency is related to the magnetic field influencing the protons. If all the protons experience the same magnetic field B_0, then only one frequency would be present within the FID. In reality, the magnetic field varies throughout the magnet and inside the patient, and thus the MR signal contains many frequencies varying as a function of time following the RF pulse. It is easier to examine such a multicomponent signal in terms of frequency rather than of time. The conversion of the signal amplitudes from a function of time to a function of frequency is accomplished using a mathematical operation called the Fourier transformation. In the frequency presentation or frequency domain spectrum, the MR signal is mapped according to its frequency relative to a reference frequency, typically the transmitter frequency ω_{TR}. For systems using quadrature detectors (see Chapter 13), ω_{TR} is centered in the display with frequencies higher and lower than ω_{TR} located to the left and right, respectively (Figure 2.3b). The frequency domain thus allows a simple way to examine the magnetic environment that a proton experiences.

Since the proton precession is continuous, the MR signal is continuous or analog in nature. However, postprocessing techniques such as Fourier transformation requires a digital representation of the signal. To produce a digital version, the FID signal is measured or sampled using an analog-to-digital

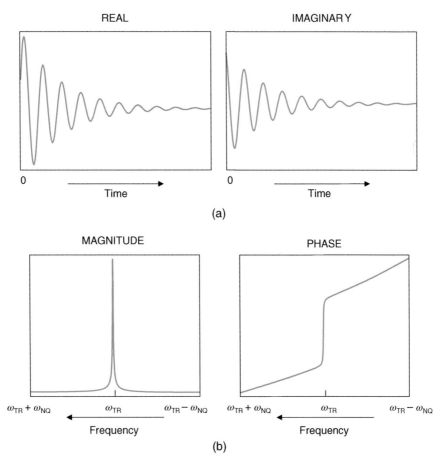

Figure 2.3 (a) Free induction decay, real and imaginary. The response of the net magnetization M to an RF pulse as a function of time is known as the free induction decay (FID). Its amplitude is proportional to the amount of transverse magnetization generated by the pulse. The FID is maximized when using a 90° excitation pulse. (b) Fourier transformation of (a), magnitude and phase. The Fourier transformation is used to convert the digital version of the MR signal (FID) from a function of time to a function of frequency. Signals measured with a quadrature detector are displayed with the transmitter (reference) frequency ω_{TR} in the middle of the display. The Nyquist frequencies ω_{NQ} below and above ω_{TR} are the minimum and maximum frequencies of the frequency display, respectively. For historical reasons, frequencies are plotted with lower frequencies on the right side and higher frequencies on the left side of the display.

converter (ADC). In most instances, the resonant frequencies of protons are greater than many ADCs can process. For this reason, a phase-coherent difference signal is generated based on the frequency and phase of the input RF pulse; that is, the signal actually digitized is the measured signal relative to ω_{TR}. This is equivalent to examining the signal in a frame of reference rotating at ω_{TR}. Under normal conditions, this so-called demodulated signal is digitized for

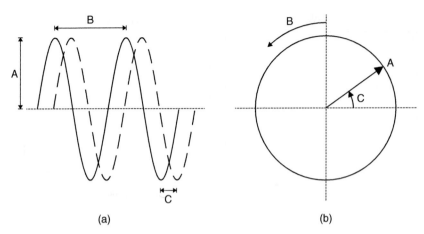

(a)   (b)

Figure 2.4 Planar (a) and circular (b) representations of a time-varying wave. The amplitude (A) is the maximum deviation of the wave from its mean value. The period (B) is the time required for completion of one complete cycle of the wave. The frequency of the wave is the reciprocal of the period. The phase or phase angle of the wave (C) describes the shift in the wave relative to a reference (a second wave for the planar representation, horizontal axis for circular representation). The two plane waves displayed in (a) have the same amplitude and period (frequency) but have a phase difference of $\pi/4$, or 90°.

a predetermined time known as the sampling time and with a user-selectable number of data points. In such a situation, there will be a maximum frequency, known as the Nyquist frequency ω_{NQ}, that can be accurately measured:

$$\omega_{NQ} = \text{(Total number of data points)}/2 \ * \ \text{(Total sampling time)} \qquad (2.2)$$

In MR, the Nyquist frequency typically ranges from 500 to 500,000 Hz, depending on the combination of sampling time and number of data points. To exclude frequencies greater than the Nyquist limit from the signal, a filter known as a low pass filter is used prior to digitization. Frequencies excluded by the low pass filter are usually noise, so that filtering provides a method for improving the signal-to-noise ratio (SNR) for the measurement. The optimum SNR is usually obtained by increasing the sampling time to match the Nyquist frequency and low pass filter width for the particular measurement conditions. For quadrature detection systems typically used in MR, the total receiver bandwidth is $2 * \omega_{NQ}$ centered about ω_{TR} (Figure 2.3b).

2.3 Chemical shift

The specific frequency that a proton absorbs is dependent on magnetic fields arising from two sources. One is the applied magnetic field B_0. The other one is molecular in origin and produces the chemical shift. In patients, the bulk of the hydrogen MR signals arise from two sources, water and fat. Water has two hydrogen atoms bonded to one oxygen atom while fat is heterogeneous in nature, with many hydrogen atoms bonded to a long chain carbon framework (typically 10–18 carbon atoms in length). Because of its different molecular environment, a water proton has a different local magnetic field than a fat proton. This local field difference is known as chemical shielding and produces a magnetic field variation that is proportional to the main magnetic field B_0:

$$B_i = B_0(1 - \sigma_i) \tag{2.3}$$

where B_i is the magnetic field and σ_i is the shielding term for proton i. Chemical shielding produces different resonant frequencies for fat and water protons under the influence of the same main magnetic field. Because the shielding term is typically small ($\sim 10^{-4}$–10^{-6}), these frequency differences are very small. It is more practical to analyze the frequencies using these differences rather than using absolute terms. A convenient scale to express frequency differences is the ppm scale, which is the resonant frequency of the proton of interest relative to a reference frequency:

$$\omega_{i(ppm)} = (\omega_{i(Hz)} - \omega_{ref})/\omega_{ref} \tag{2.4}$$

Frequency differences expressed in this form are known as chemical shifts. While the choice of ω_{ref} is arbitrary, a convenient choice is ω_{TR}. The primary advantage of the ppm scale is that frequency differences are independent of B_0. For fat and water, the difference in chemical shifts at all field strengths is approximately 3.5 ppm, with fat at a lower frequency. At 1.5 T, this difference is 220 Hz, while at 3.0 T, it is 450 Hz (Figure 2.5).

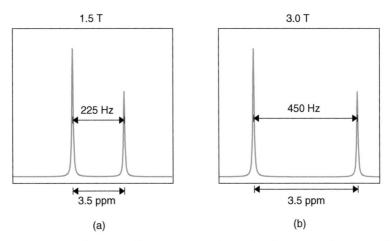

Figure 2.5 Spectrum of water and fat at 1.5 T (a) and 3.0 T (b). The resonant frequencies for water and fat are separated by approximately 3.5 ppm, which corresponds to an absolute frequency difference of 220 Hz for a 1.5 T magnetic field (63 MHz) or 450 Hz at a magnetic field of 3.0 T (126 MHz).

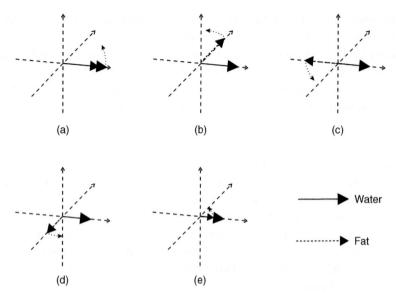

Figure 2.6 Precession of fat and water protons. Because of the 3.5 ppm frequency difference, a fat proton precesses at a slower frequency than does a water proton. In a rotating frame at the water resonant frequency, the fat proton cycles in and out of phase with the water proton. Following the excitation pulse, the two protons are in phase (a). After a short time, they will be 90° out of phase (b), then 180° out of phase (c, also called "opposed phase"). Then −90° out of phase (d) and back in phase (e). The contribution of fat to the total signal fluctuates and depends on when the signal is detected. At 1.5 T, the in-phase times are 0 ms (a), 4.5 ms (e), 9 ms and so on (not shown), while the opposed-phase times are 2.25 ms (c), 6.7 ms and so on (not shown). At 3.0 T, the times are one half of the times at 1.5 T.

The chemical shift difference between fat and water can be visualized in the rotating frame. A 150 Hz difference in frequency means that the fat resonance precesses slower than the water resonance by 6.7 ms per cycle (1/150 Hz). The fat resonance will align with or be in phase with the water resonance every 6.7 ms at 1.0 T. For a 1.5 T MR system, the same cycling will occur every 4.5 ms (1/220 Hz) and every 2.25 ms for a 3.0 T system (Figure 2.6). The 3.5 ppm chemical shift difference mentioned previously is an approximate difference. The fat resonance signal is a composite from all the protons within the fat molecule. The particular chemical composition (e.g., saturated versus unsaturated hydrocarbon chain, length of hydrocarbon chain) determines the exact resonant frequency for this composite signal. The 3.5 ppm difference applies to the majority of fatty tissues found in the body. Chemical shift differences between protons in different molecular environments provide the basis for MR spectroscopy, which is described in more detail in Chapter 13.

CHAPTER 3

Relaxation

As mentioned in Chapter 2, the MR measurement can be analyzed in terms of energy transfer. The process by which the protons release the energy that they absorbed from the RF pulse is known as relaxation. Relaxation is a fundamental aspect of MR, as essential as energy absorption, and provides the primary mechanism for image contrast as discussed in Chapter 6. In resonance absorption, RF energy is absorbed by the protons only when it is broadcast at the correct frequency. The additional energy disturbs the equilibrium arrangement of spins parallel and antiparallel to B_0. Following excitation, relaxation occurs in which the protons release this added energy and return to their original configuration through naturally occurring processes. It is a time-dependent process and is characterized by a rate constant known as the relaxation time. Although it is individual protons that absorb the energy, relaxation times are measured for an entire sample of spins and are statistical or average quantities. Relaxation times are measured for gray matter or cerebrospinal fluid as bulk samples rather than for the individual water or fat molecules within the organs. Two relaxation times can be measured, known as *T1* and *T2*. While both times measure the spontaneous energy transfer by an excited proton, they differ in the final disposition of the energy.

3.1 *T1* relaxation and saturation

 The relaxation time *T1* is the time required for the *z* component of **M** to return to 63% of its original value following an excitation pulse. It is also known as the spin-lattice relaxation time or longitudinal relaxation time. Recall from Chapter 2 that M_0 is parallel to B_0 at equilibrium and that energy absorption will rotate M_0 into the transverse plane. *T1* relaxation provides the mechanism by which the protons give up their energy to return to their original orientation. If a 90° pulse is applied to a sample, M_0 will rotate as illustrated in Figure 2.2, and there will be no longitudinal magnetization present following the pulse. As time goes on, a return of the longitudinal magnetization will be observed as

MRI Basic Principles and Applications, Fifth Edition.
Brian M. Dale, Mark A. Brown and Richard C. Semelka.
© 2015 John Wiley & Sons, Ltd. Published 2015 by John Wiley & Sons, Ltd.

the protons release their energy (Figure 3.1). This return of magnetization typically follows an exponential growth process, with *T1* being the time constant describing the rate of growth:

$$M(\tau) = M_0(1 - e^{-\tau/T1})$$ (3.1)

where τ is the time following the RF pulse. *T1* relaxation times in tissues are relatively slow, with values ranging from a few milliseconds to several seconds. After 3 *T1* time periods, **M** will have returned to 95% of its value prior to the excitation pulse, **M_0**. The term spin-lattice refers to the fact that the excited proton ("spin") transfers its energy to its surroundings ("lattice") rather than to another proton. The energy no longer contributes to spin excitation.

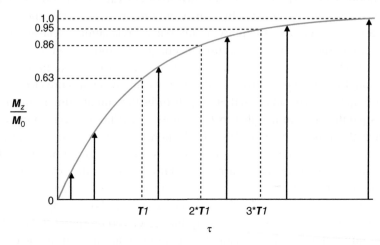

Figure 3.1 *T1* relaxation curve. Immediately following a 90° RF pulse, there is no longitudinal magnetization. A short time later, longitudinal magnetization will be observed as the protons release their energy through *T1* relaxation. Gradually, as more protons release their energy, a larger fraction of **M_z** is reestablished. Eventually, **M_0** will be restored completely. The change of **M_z**/**M_0** with time τ follows an exponential growth process as described by equation (3.1). The time constant for this process is *T1*, the spin-lattice relaxation time, and is the time when **M_z** has returned to 63% of its original value.

In a modern MR experiment, pulsed RF energy is applied to the protons repeatedly with a delay time between the pulses. This time between pulses allows the excited protons to give up the absorbed energy (*T1* relaxation). As the protons give up this energy to their surroundings, the population difference (spin up versus spin down) is reestablished so that net absorption can reoccur after the next pulse. In the macroscopic picture, **M** returns toward its initial value M_0 as more energy is dissipated. Since **M** is the ultimate source of the MR signal, the more energy dissipated, the more signal is generated following the next RF pulse.

For practical reasons, the time between successive RF pulses is usually insufficient for complete *T1* relaxation so that **M** will not be completely restored to M_0. Application of a second RF pulse prior to complete relaxation will rotate **M** into the transverse plane, but with a smaller magnitude than following the first RF pulse. The following experiment describes the situation (Figure 3.2):

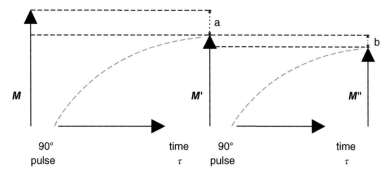

Figure 3.2 Following a 90° RF pulse, longitudinal magnetization is regenerated through *T1* relaxation. If the time between successive RF pulses τ is insufficient for complete recovery of *M*, only *M'* will be present at the time of the next RF pulse (a). If time τ elapses again, only *M''* will be present (b). *M''* will be smaller than *M'*, but the difference will be less than the difference between *M* and *M'*.

1 A 90° RF pulse is applied. *M* is rotated into the transverse plane.
2 A time τ elapses, insufficient for complete *T1* relaxation. The longitudinal magnetization at the end of τ, *M'*, is less than in step 1.
3 A second 90° RF pulse is applied. *M'* is rotated into the transverse plane.
4 After a second time τ elapses, *M''* is produced. It is smaller in magnitude than *M'*, but the difference is less than the difference between *M* and *M'*.

 Following a few repetitions, *M* returns to the same magnitude prior to each RF pulse; that is, *M* achieves a steady-state value. In general, this steady-state value depends on five parameters:
1 The main magnetic field strength B_0. The larger the value for B_0, the larger is M.
2 The number of protons producing *M* (per unit volume of tissue, known as the proton density).
3 The amount of energy absorbed by the protons (the pulse angle or flip angle).
4 The rate of RF pulse application (time τ).
5 The efficiency of the protons in giving up their energy (*T1* relaxation time).

For many MRI experiments such as standard spin echo and gradient echo imaging, a steady state of *M* is present because multiple RF pulses are applied and the repetition time *TR* between the pulses is nearly always less than sufficient for complete relaxation. To produce this steady state prior to data collection, additional RF pulses are applied to the tissue immediately prior to the main imaging pulses. These extra RF pulses are known as preparatory pulses or dummy pulses because the generated signals are usually ignored. These preparatory pulses ensure that *M* has the same magnitude prior to every measurement during the scan.

The rate of RF pulse application and the efficiency of energy transfer must have the proper balance. Suppose the RF energy is applied faster than *T1* relaxation can occur. A comparison of the microscopic and macroscopic pictures is useful at this point. In the microscopic picture, the protons in the lower energy level absorb the RF energy and the protons in the upper energy level are stimulated to emit their energy. As more energy is transmitted, the proton populations of the two levels will gradually equalize. When this equalization occurs, no further net absorption of energy is possible, a condition known as saturation (Figure 3.3). In the macroscopic picture, *M* will rotate continuously but gradually get smaller in magnitude until it disappears as the net population difference approaches zero. Since there is no net magnetization, there will be no coherence of proton motion in the transverse plane and thus no signal is produced. This condition is known as saturation. There is a limited amount of energy that a collection of protons can absorb before they become saturated. In a conventional MR measurement, each tissue will experience different amounts of saturation, due to their different *T1* relaxation times. As a result, the contribution of a tissue to *M* will differ, as will its maximum potential signal.

As mentioned earlier, spin-lattice relaxation measures the rate of energy transfer from an excited proton to its surroundings. The key to this energy transfer is the presence of some type of molecular motion (e.g., vibration, rotation) of the lattice in the vicinity of the excited proton with an intrinsic frequency, ω_L, that matches the resonant frequency, ω_0. The closer ω_0 is to ω_L, the more readily the motion absorbs the energy and the more frequently this energy transfer occurs, allowing the collection of protons to return to its equilibrium configuration sooner. In tissues, the nature of the protein molecular structure and any metal ions that may be present have a pronounced effect on the particular ω_L. Metals ions such as iron or manganese can have significant magnetic moments that may influence the local environment. While the particular protein structures are different for many tissues, the molecular rotation or tumbling of most proteins typically have ω_L of approximately 1 MHz. Therefore, at lower resonant frequencies (lower B_0), there is a better match

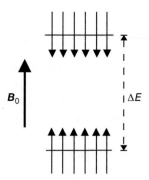

Figure 3.3 Saturation. If RF pulses are applied faster than the *T1* relaxation processes can dissipate the energy, the spin populations equalize between the two energy levels. As a result, there is no difference in the number of spins and no net magnetization.

between ω_L and ω_0. This enables a more efficient energy transfer to occur and thus *T1* is shorter. This is the basis for the frequency dependence of *T1*; namely, *T1* decreases with decreasing strength of the magnetic field. This is also the reason that a larger B_0 does not necessarily translate to a greater signal, as saturation is more prevalent due to the longer *T1* times.

3.2 *T2* relaxation, *T2** relaxation, and spin echoes

The relaxation time *T2* is the time required for the transverse component of **M** to decay to 37% of its initial value through irreversible processes. It is also known as the spin–spin relaxation time or transverse relaxation time. Recall from Chapter 1 that M_0 is oriented only along the z (B_0) axis at equilibrium and that no portion of M_0 is in the xy plane. The coherence is entirely longitudinal or parallel to B_0. Absorption of energy from a 90° RF pulse as in Figure 2.2 causes M_0 to rotate entirely into the xy plane, so that the coherence is in the transverse plane at the end of the pulse. As time elapses, this coherence disappears while at the same time the protons release their energy and reorient themselves along B_0. This disappearing coherence produces the FID described in Chapter 2. As this coherence disappears, the value of **M** in the xy plane decreases toward 0. *T2* or *T2** relaxation is the process by which this transverse magnetization is lost.

A comparison of the microscopic and macroscopic pictures provides additional insight. At the end of the 90° RF pulse, when the protons have absorbed energy and **M** is oriented in the transverse plane, each proton precesses at the same frequency ω_0 and is synchronized at the same point or phase of its precessional cycle. Since a nearby proton of the same type will have the same molecular environment and the same ω_0, it can readily absorb the energy that is being released by its neighbor. Spin–spin relaxation refers to this energy transfer from an excited proton to another nearby proton (Figure 3.4). The absorbed energy remains as spin excitation

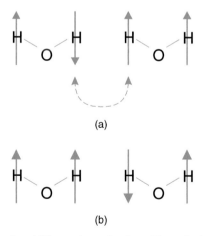

(a)

(b)

Figure 3.4 Spin–spin relaxation. (a) Two water molecules, with one hydrogen atom on one molecule having absorbed RF energy and being excited (spin down). (b) If the molecules are in close proximity, the energy can be transferred from the first water molecule to a hydrogen atom on the second water molecule.

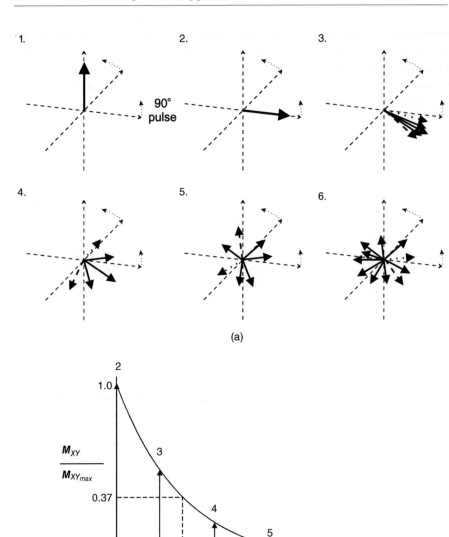

(a)

(b)

Figure 3.5 (a) A rotating frame slower than ω_0 is assumed for this figure. Net magnetization $\boldsymbol{M}$ (arrow) is oriented parallel to $\boldsymbol{B}_0$ (not shown) prior to an RF pulse (1). Following a 90° RF pulse, the spins precess initially in phase in the transverse plane (2). Due to inter-and intramolecular interactions, the spins begin to precess at different frequencies (dashed arrow, faster; dotted arrow, slower) and become asynchronous with each other (3). As more time elapses (4,5), the transverse coherence becomes smaller until there is complete randomness of the transverse components and no coherence (6). (b) Plot of relative $\boldsymbol{M}_{XY}$ component as a function of time. The numbers correspond to the expected $\boldsymbol{M}_{XY}$ component from (a). The change in $\boldsymbol{M}_{XY}/\boldsymbol{M}_{XY\,max}$ with time follows an exponential decay process as described by equation (3.3). The time constant for this process is the spin-spin relaxation time $T2^*$ and is the time when $\boldsymbol{M}_{XY}$ has decayed to 37% of its original value.

rather than being transferred to the surroundings as in *T1* relaxation. This proton–proton energy transfer can occur many times as long as the protons are in close proximity and remain at the same ω_0. Intermolecular and intramolecular interactions such as vibrations or rotations cause transient fluctuations in the magnetic field and thus cause ω_0 to fluctuate. This fluctuation produces a gradual, irreversible loss of phase coherence to the spins as they exchange the energy and reduce the magnitude of the transverse magnetization and the generated signal (Figure 3.5). *T2* is the time when the transverse magnetization is 37% of its value immediately after the 90° pulse when this irreversible process is the only cause for the loss of coherence. As more time elapses, this transverse coherence completely disappears, only to reform in the longitudinal direction as *T1* relaxation occurs. This dephasing time *T2* is always less than or equal to *T1*.

There are several potential causes for a loss of transverse coherence to M. One is the molecular motions of the adjacent spins due to vibrations or rotations. This irreversible movement is responsible for spin–spin relaxation or the true *T2*. Another cause arises from the fact that a proton never experiences a magnetic field that is 100% uniform or homogeneous in value. As the proton precesses, it experiences a fluctuating local magnetic field, causing a change in ω_0 and a loss in transverse phase coherence. This nonuniformity in B_0 comes from three sources:

1 Main field inhomogeneity. There is always some degree of nonuniformity to B_0 due to imperfections in magnet manufacturing, interactions with nearby building walls, or other sources of metal. This field distortion is constant during the measurement time.

2 Sample-induced inhomogeneity. Differences in the magnetic susceptibility or degree of magnetic polarization of adjacent tissues (e.g., bone, air) will distort the local magnetic field near the interface between the different tissues. Provided there is no motion of the sample, this inhomogeneity is also of constant magnitude and is present as long as the patient is present within the magnet.

3 Imaging gradients. As discussed in Chapter 4, the technique used for spatial localization generates a magnetic field inhomogeneity that induces proton dephasing. This inhomogeneity is transient during the measurement.

 The contributions of the imaging gradients may be eliminated as a source of dephasing through proper design of the measurement process, as described in Chapter 4. The other sources contribute to the total transverse relaxation time, *T2**:

$$1/T2^* = 1/T2 + 1/T2_M + 1/T2_{MS} \tag{3.2}$$

where $T2_M$ is the dephasing time due to the main field inhomogeneity and $T2_{MS}$ is the dephasing time due to the magnetic susceptibility differences. The decay of the transverse magnetization following a 90° RF pulse, the FID, follows an approximately exponential process with the time constant of $T2^*$ rather than just $T2$:

$$M_{XY}(t) = M_{XY\,max}e^{-t/T2^*}$$

(3.3)

where $M_{XY\,max}$ is the transverse magnetization M_{XY} immediately following the excitation pulse. For most tissues or liquids, $T2_M$ is the major factor in determining $T2^*$, while for tissue with significant iron deposits or air-filled cavities, $T2_{MS}$ dominates $T2^*$.

Some sources of proton dephasing can be reversed by the application of a 180° RF pulse, which is described by the following sequence of events (Figure 3.6):

1 A 90° RF pulse.
2 A short delay of time t.
3 A 180° RF pulse.
4 A second time delay t.

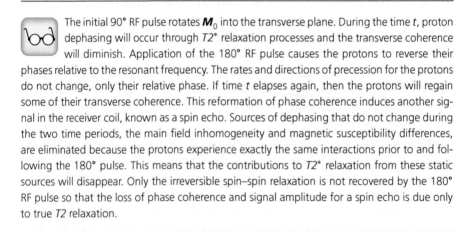

The initial 90° RF pulse rotates M_0 into the transverse plane. During the time t, proton dephasing will occur through $T2^*$ relaxation processes and the transverse coherence will diminish. Application of the 180° RF pulse causes the protons to reverse their phases relative to the resonant frequency. The rates and directions of precession for the protons do not change, only their relative phase. If time t elapses again, then the protons will regain some of their transverse coherence. This reformation of phase coherence induces another signal in the receiver coil, known as a spin echo. Sources of dephasing that do not change during the two time periods, the main field inhomogeneity and magnetic susceptibility differences, are eliminated because the protons experience exactly the same interactions prior to and following the 180° pulse. This means that the contributions to $T2^*$ relaxation from these static sources will disappear. Only the irreversible spin–spin relaxation is not recovered by the 180° RF pulse so that the loss of phase coherence and signal amplitude for a spin echo is due only to true $T2$ relaxation.

Following the echo formation, the protons continue to precess and dephase a second time as the sources of dephasing continue to affect them. Application of a second 180° RF pulse again reverses the proton phases and generates another coherence to the protons, producing another spin echo. This second echo differs from the first echo by the increased amount of $T2$ relaxation contributing to the signal loss. This process of spin echo formation by 180° RF pulses can be repeated as many times as desired, until $T2$ relaxation completely dephases the protons. The use of multiple 180° pulses maintains phase coherence to the protons longer than the use of a single 180° RF pulse because of the significant dephasing that the field inhomogeneity induces over very short time periods.

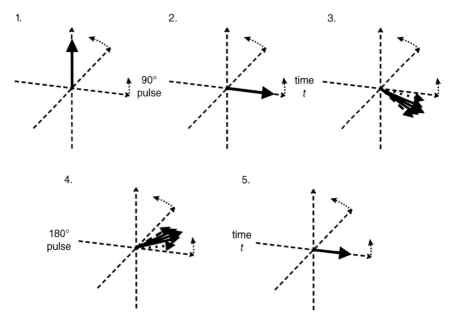

Figure 3.6 A rotation frame slower than ω_0 is assumed for this figure. Net magnetization M (arrow) is oriented parallel to B_0 (not shown) prior to an RF pulse (1). Application of a 90° RF pulse rotates M into the transverse plane (2). Due to the $T2^*$ relaxation processes, the protons become asynchronous with each other during time t (3). Application of a 180° RF pulse causes the protons to reverse their phase relative to the transmitter phase. The protons that precessed most rapidly are farthest behind (dashed arrow), while the slowest protons are in front (dotted arrow) (4). Allowing time t to elapse again allows the protons to regain their phase coherence in the transverse plane (5), generating a signal in the receiver coil known as a spin echo. The loss in magnitude of the reformed coherence relative to the original coherence (2) is due to irreversible processes (i.e., true spin–spin or T2 relaxation). Equation (3.3) describes the decay of M_{XY} if T2 is used instead of $T2^*$.

One important difference between $T1$ and $T2$ relaxation is in the influence of B_0. As mentioned earlier, $T1$ is very sensitive to B_0, with longer $T1$ times measured for a tissue at higher B_0. $T2$ is relatively insensitive to B_0 at the relatively large field strengths currently used in MRI. Only at very low B_0 (less than 0.05 T) will there be significant changes in $T2$. The other components of $T2^*$, $T2_M$ and $T2_{MS}$ become more prominent at higher B_0. Good magnetic field uniformity is more difficult to generate at high magnetic fields, so that $T2_M$ will be shorter. Greater B_0 will also cause greater differences in M_0 between two tissues with different magnetic susceptibilities, producing shorter $T2_{MS}$. The result is that T2-weighted techniques will see little sensitivity to B_0 while $T2^*$-weighted techniques will show greater signal differences at higher B_0.

CHAPTER 4

Principles of magnetic resonance imaging – 1

Chapter 2 described the relationship between the frequency of energy that a proton absorbs and the magnetic field strength that it experiences. MRI uses this field dependence to localize these proton frequencies to different regions of space. This idea of using the field dependence to spatially localize the protons earned the 2003 Nobel Prize in Physiology or Medicine for Paul Lauterbur and Sir Peter Mansfield, and helped transform MR from a niche industry serving research labs into a multibillion-dollar industry serving hospitals worldwide.

4.1 Gradient fields

In MRI, the magnetic field is made spatially dependent through the application of magnetic field gradients. These gradients are relatively small perturbations superimposed on the main magnetic field B_0, with a typical imaging gradient producing a total field variation of less than 1%. They are also linear perturbations to B_0, so that the exact magnetic field is linearly dependent on the location inside the magnet:

$$B_i = B_0 + G_T \otimes r_i \qquad (4.1)$$

where B_i is the magnetic field at location r_i and G_T is the total gradient amplitude, mathematically represented as a tensor. Gradients are also applied for short periods of time during a scan and are referred to as gradient pulses.

In clinical MRI, the magnetic field gradients that are used produce linear variations primarily in one direction only, so that the tensor product in equation 4.1 can be reduced to a vector representation. Each gradient is centered around a point in the center of the magnet known as an isocenter. Variations to one side of the isocenter will have total magnetic field values B_i greater than that at the isocenter (B_0) while locations on the other side will have B_i less than B_0. The gradient amplitude is the slope of the line, as illustrated in Figure 4.1.

MRI Basic Principles and Applications, Fifth Edition.
Brian M. Dale, Mark A. Brown and Richard C. Semelka.
© 2015 John Wiley & Sons, Ltd. Published 2015 by John Wiley & Sons, Ltd.

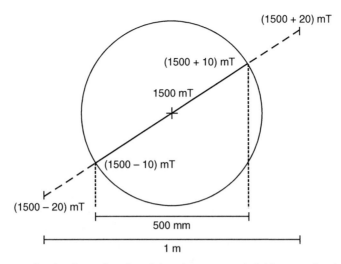

Figure 4.1 A gradient is a linear distortion of the primary magnetic field, centered at the magnet isocenter. A 40 mT m⁻¹ gradient superimposed on a 1.5 T magnet field will produce a total magnetic field variation of 1480 to 1520 mT. For a 500 mm distance, the variation will be 1490 to 1510 mT.

In the direction perpendicular or normal to the gradient, B_i will be constant. In other words, the presence of a gradient will produce planes of constant B_i, with the value of B_i variation dependent on its location. The direction of B_i variation is perpendicular or normal to the surface of the plane. Three physical gradients are used, one in each of the $x, y,$ and z directions. Each one is assigned, through the operating software, to one or more of the three "logical" or functional gradients required to obtain an image: slice selection, readout or frequency encoding, and phase encoding. The particular pairing of physical and logical gradients is somewhat arbitrary and depends on the acquisition parameters and patient positioning as well as the choice of physical directions by the manufacturer. The only requirement is that the three logical directions must be mutually perpendicular. The combination of gradient pulses, RF pulses, data sampling periods, and the timing between each of them that are used to acquire an image is known as a pulse sequence.

The presence of linear magnetic field gradients requires an expanded version of the Larmor equation given in equation (1.1):

$$\omega_i = \gamma(B_0 + \mathbf{G} \bullet \mathbf{r}_i) \tag{4.2}$$

where ω_i is the frequency of the proton at position $\mathbf{r}_i$ and $\mathbf{G}$ is a vector representing the total gradient amplitude and direction. The units of measure for G are expressed in millitesla per meter (mT m⁻¹) or gauss per centimeter (G cm⁻¹), where 1 G cm⁻¹ = 10 mT m⁻¹. Equation 4.2 states that, in the presence of a gradient field, each proton will resonate at a unique frequency that depends on its exact position within the gradient field. The MR image is simply a frequency and phase map of the protons generated by unique magnetic fields at each point throughout the image. The displayed image consists of digital picture elements (pixels) that represent volume elements (voxels) of tissue. The pixel intensity is related to the number of protons contained within the voxel weighted by the tissue characteristics, like *T1* and *T2* relaxation times, for the tissues within the voxel according to the pulse sequence utilized.

4.2 Slice selection

The initial step in MRI is the localization of the RF excitation to a region of space, which is accomplished through the use of frequency-selective excitation in conjunction with a gradient known as the slice selection gradient, G_{SS}. The gradient direction (x, y, z or a combination) determines the slice orientation while the gradient amplitude together with certain RF pulse characteristics determine both the slice thickness and slice position. A frequency-selective RF pulse has two key features: a central frequency and a narrow range or bandwidth of frequencies (typically 1–2 kHz) (see Chapter 5 for a more detailed description of selective pulses). When such a pulse is broadcast in the presence of the slice selection gradient, a narrow region of tissue achieves the resonance condition (equation 4.2) and absorbs the RF energy. The duration of the RF pulse and its amplitude determines the amount of resulting rotation of **M** (e.g., 90°, 180°). The central frequency of the pulse determines the particular location excited by the pulse when the slice selection gradient is present. Different slice positions are achieved by changing

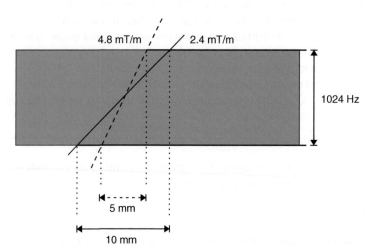

Figure 4.2 For a given range (bandwidth) of frequencies included in the RF pulse, the slice thickness desired is determined by the slice-selection gradient amplitude. The user interface typically allows variation of the slice thickness, which is achieved by increasing or decreasing the slice-selection gradient amplitude, as appropriate.

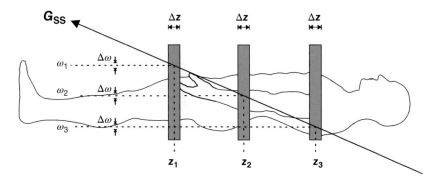

Figure 4.3 Slice-selection process. In the presence of a gradient (G_{SS}), the total magnetic field that a proton experiences and its resulting resonant frequency depend on its position according to equation 4.2. Tissue located at position z_i will absorb RF energy broadcast with a center frequency ω_i. Each position will have a unique resonant frequency. The slice thickness Δz is determined by the amplitude (magnitude) of G_{SS} and by the bandwidth of transmitted frequencies $\Delta\omega$.

the central frequency. The slice thickness is determined by the gradient amplitude G_{SS} and the bandwidth of frequencies $\Delta\omega_{SS}$ incorporated into the RF pulse:

$$\Delta\omega_{SS} = \gamma(G_{SS} * \text{Thickness}) \tag{4.3}$$

Typically, $\Delta\omega_{SS}$ is fixed for a given pulse sequence, so that the slice thickness is changed by modifying the amplitude of G_{SS} (Figure 4.2). Thinner slices require larger G_{SS}. Once G_{SS} is determined by the slice thickness, the central frequency is calculated using equation 4.2 to bring the desired location into resonance. Multislice imaging, the most commonly used approach for MRI, uses the same G_{SS} but a unique RF pulse during excitation for each slice. The RF pulse for each slice has the same bandwidth but a different central frequency, thereby exciting a different region of tissue (Figure 4.3).

The slice orientation is determined by the particular physical gradient or gradients defined as the logical slice selection gradient. The slice orientation is defined so that the gradient orientation is perpendicular or normal to the surface of the slice, so that every proton within the slice experiences the same total magnetic field (to within the bandwidth) regardless of its position within the slice. Orthogonal slices are those in which only the x,y, or z gradient is used as the slice selection gradient. Oblique slices, those not in one of the principal directions, are obtained by applying more than one physical gradient when the RF pulse is broadcast. The total gradient amplitude, whether from one, two, or three physical gradients, determines the slice thickness as shown in equation 4.3. When images are viewed on the monitor or film, the slice selection direction is always perpendicular to the surface; that is, hidden from the viewer (Figure 4.4).

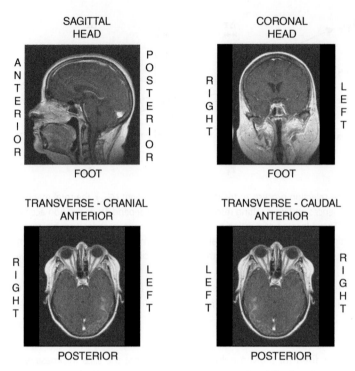

Figure 4.4 Images in standard slice orientations: sagittal, coronal, and transverse or axial. For transverse images, two view directions are possible: cranial and caudal. Image annotations are based on patient axes.

4.3 Readout or frequency encoding

The signal detection portion of the MRI measurement is known as Readout or Frequency Encoding. The readout process differentiates MRI from MR spectroscopy, the other type of MR experiment (see Chapter 13). In an imaging pulse sequence, the MR signal is always detected in the presence of a gradient known as the readout gradient G_{RO}, which produces one of the spatial dimensions of the image. A typical pulse sequence uses some form of excitation, such as a 90° slice-selective pulse, to excite a particular region of tissue. Following excitation, the net magnetization within the slice is oriented transverse to B_0 and will precess with frequency ω_0. T2* processes induce dephasing of this transverse magnetization (see Chapter 3). This dephasing can be partially reversed to form an echo by the application of a 180° RF pulse, a gradient pulse, or both. As the echo is forming, the readout gradient is applied perpendicular to the slice direction. Under the influence of this new gradient field, the protons precess at different frequencies depending on their position within it, in accordance with equation 4.2. Each of these frequencies is superimposed into the echo. At the desired time, the echo signal is measured by the receiver coil and digitized for later Fourier transformation. The magnitude of the readout gradient G_{RO} and the frequency that is detected enable the corresponding position of the proton to be determined (Figure 4.5).

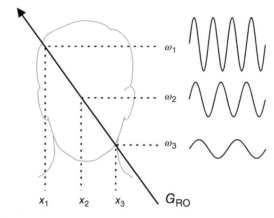

Figure 4.5 Readout process. Following excitation, each spin within the excited volume (slice) precesses at the same frequency. During detection of the echo, a gradient (G_{RO}) is applied, causing a variation in the frequencies for the spins generating the echo signal. The frequency of precession ω_i for each spin depends on its position x_i according to equation 4.2. Frequencies measured from the echo are mapped to the corresponding position.

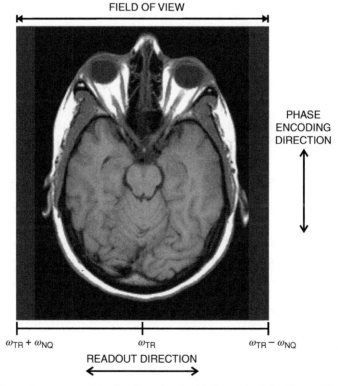

Figure 4.6 In any image, one of the directions visualized is the readout direction and the other is the phase-encoding direction. A proton located at the edge of the FOV in the readout direction precesses at the Nyquist frequency ω_{NQ} above or below the transmitter frequency ω_{TR}. Changing the FOV of the image changes the spatial resolution (millimeters per pixel) but not the frequency resolution (hertz per pixel).

The magnitude of G_{RO} is determined by two user-definable parameters: the field of view (FOV) in the readout direction, FOV_{RO}, and the Nyquist frequency ω_{NQ} for the image, often referred to as the receiver bandwidth (equation (2.2)). This relationship is expressed in the following equation:

$$\Delta\omega_{RO} = 2 * \omega_{NQ} = \gamma(G_{RO} * FOV_{RO}) \tag{4.4}$$

where $\Delta\omega_{RO}$ is the total range of frequencies in the image. G_{RO} is chosen so that protons located at the edge of FOV_{RO} precess at the Nyquist frequency above the transmitter frequency ω_{TR} for the image (Figure 4.6). Smaller FOV_{RO} values can be achieved by increasing G_{RO}, keeping the Nyquist frequency and thus the total frequency bandwidth constant (Figure 4.7).

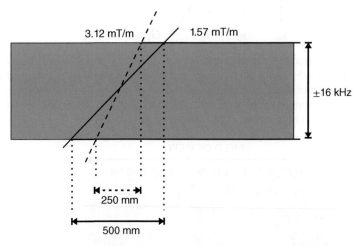

Figure 4.7 For a given range (bandwidth) of frequencies that are measured in the signal, the desired *FOV* is determined by the readout gradient amplitude. The user interface typically allows variation of the *FOV*, which is achieved by increasing or decreasing the readout gradient amplitude, as appropriate.

In an MR image, the resolution may be expressed in one of two ways: the spatial resolution and the frequency resolution. The spatial resolution, expressed as the voxel size with units of mm/pixel, is derived from two user parameters, FOV_{RO} and the number of readout sample points in the acquisition matrix, N_{RO}:

$$VOX_{RO} = FOV_{RO}/N_{RO} \tag{4.5}$$

The frequency resolution, with units of Hz/pixel, is based on N_{RO} and $\Delta\omega_{RO}$ for the image:

$$\text{Pixel bandwidth} = \Delta\omega_{RO}/N_{RO} = 2 * \omega_{NQ}/N_{RO} \tag{4.6}$$

It is possible to improve the frequency resolution for the measurement independent of the spatial resolution by increasing the total sampling time used to measure the signal. This reduces the Nyquist frequency for the image and the background noise contributing to the measurement. In order to maintain the correct spatial resolution within the image, G_{RO} is reduced, in accordance with equation 4.4.

4.4 Phase encoding

The third direction in an MR image is the phase encoding direction. It is visualized along with the readout direction in a two-dimensional (2D) image (see Figure 4.5). The phase encoding gradient, G_{PE}, is perpendicular to both G_{SS} and G_{RO} and is the only gradient that changes amplitude during the data acquisition loop of a standard 2D imaging sequence. Any signal variation detected from one acquisition to the next is assumed to be caused by the influence of G_{PE} during the measurement.

The principle of phase encoding is based on the fact that the proton precession is periodic in nature. Prior to the application of G_{PE}, a proton within a slice precesses at the base frequency ω_0. In the presence of G_{PE}, its precessional frequency increases or decreases along the PE direction according to equation 4.2. Once G_{PE} is turned off, the proton precession returns to its original frequency, but is ahead or behind in phase relative to its previous state. This phase difference alters the amplitude that the proton will contribute to the final signal. The amount of induced phase change depends on the magnitude and

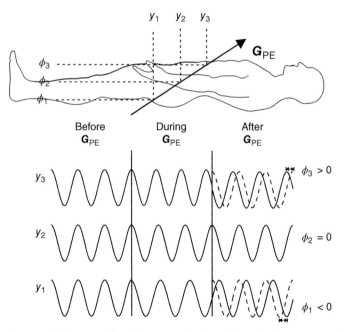

Figure 4.8 Concept of phase encoding. Prior to application of G_{PE}, all spins precess at the same frequency. When G_{PE} is applied, a spin increases or decreases its precessional frequency, depending on its position y_i. A spin located at $y_i = 0$ (y_2) experiences no effect from G_{PE} and no change in frequency or phase ($\phi_2 = 0$). A spin located at y_3 precesses faster while G_{PE} is applied. Once G_{PE} is turned off, the spin precesses at its original frequency but is ahead of the reference frequency (dashed curve); that is, a phase shift ϕ_3 has been induced to the proton by G_{PE}. A spin located at y_1 decreases its frequency while G_{PE} is applied. Once G_{PE} is turned off, it precesses at its original frequency but is behind the reference by a phase shift of ϕ_1.

duration of G_{PE} that the proton experienced and the proton location. Protons located at different positions in the phase encoding direction experience different amounts of phase shift for the same G_{PE} pulse (Figure 4.8). A proton located at the edge of the chosen FOV experiences the maximum amount of phase change from each phase encoding step. The MR image information is obtained by repeating the slice excitation and signal detection multiple times, each with a different amplitude of G_{PE}.

The spatial resolution in the phase encoding direction depends on two user-selectable parameters, the field of view in the phase encoding direction, FOV_{PE}, and the number of phase encoding steps in the acquisition matrix, N_{PE}. The FOV_{PE} is determined by the change in G_{PE} from one step to the next. For a proton located at the chosen FOV_{PE}, each phase encoding step induces one half-cycle (180°) of phase change relative to the previous phase encoding step, assuming a constant pulse duration (Figure 4.9). N_{PE} determines the total number of cycles of phase change ($N_{PE}/2$) produced at the edge of the FOV and thus the maximum frequency (ω_{NQ}) in the phase encoding direction for the given pulse duration. The spatial resolution in the phase encoding direction is expressed as the voxel size and is measured in mm/pixel:

$$VOX_{PE} = FOV_{PE}/N_{PE} \tag{4.7}$$

Increased resolution is obtained by reducing the FOV_{PE} or by increasing N_{PE}. The FOV reduction is accomplished by increasing the gradient amplitude change from one G_{PE} to the next.

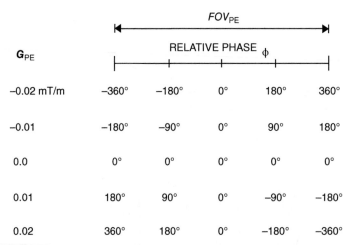

Figure 4.9 Phase-encoding process. A spin at the edge of the FOV in the phase-encoding direction undergoes 90° of phase change $\Delta\phi$ from one phase-encoding step to the next. Each point within the FOV undergoes progressively less phase change for the same gradient amplitude. A spin at isocenter never experiences any phase change. The change in gradient amplitude (0.01 mT m^{-1} in this example) from one phase-encoding step to the next is inversely proportional to the FOV ($\Delta G_{PE} \propto 1/FOV$).

Because of the two different physical processes involved, FOV_{PE} is not required to be the same as the FOV_{RO}, nor is the voxel size. The resulting pixel dimensions also need not be equal. The readout pixel size divided by the phase encoding pixel size is known as the aspect ratio between the two dimensions. An aspect ratio of 1.0 (100%) means that the pixel size is the same in both directions, a situation referred to as isotropic pixels. An aspect ratio less than 1.0 (<100%) is referred to as anisotropic pixels, with the phase encoding dimension typically larger than the readout dimension.

4.5 Sequence looping

The previous two sections described the individual steps used for spatial localization of the MR signal to a point within a slice. For most MR applications, information from many slices is measured during the scan in order to acquire images from large volumes of tissue. Several approaches are used for data acquisition that balance the desire for good spatial resolution and contrast-to-noise ratio (signal difference relative to background noise) while maintaining reasonable scan times.

In order to accomplish efficient data collection with minimal computer processing, most MRI techniques use some form of repetitive execution, which is achieved using computer instructions known as loops. This allows common instructions such as fixed amplitude gradient pulses (e.g., readout or slice selection gradient pulses) to be programmed one time yet provide a convenient method for modifying variable quantities such as phase encoding gradient amplitudes or RF pulse center frequencies.

There are several ways to differentiate measurement techniques. One method is based on the volume of tissue excited that is used to generate the signal. The most common technique is 2D multislice imaging, in which a narrow volume of tissue (typically < 10 mm) is excited by a slice-selective RF pulse and generates the echo signal. The *TR* specified by the user is the time between successive excitation pulses for a given slice. The total number of lines of data collected for each slice depends on the number of phase encoding steps, N_{PE}, and the number of signals added together for signal averaging, N_{SA}. The sequence kernel time, or minimum *TR* per slice, is the actual time required for the measurement hardware to perform all the steps necessary to acquire raw data from a single excitation, typically one line from one slice. Often, the sequence kernel time is much shorter than *TR*, allowing excitation and detection of many slices to be performed within one *TR* time period.

Traditionally, multislice scanning acquired one line of data from each slice during each *TR* time period (Figure 4.10a). This approach set a lower limit for *TR*. By subdividing the slice loop into subloops so that a subset of slices is acquired, a shorter *TR* and greater contrast control is possible. The total scan time is *TR* times the total number of lines times the number of subloops:

$$(\text{Scan time})_{\text{multislice}} = TR * N_{SA} * N_{PE} * N_{SUBLOOP} \qquad (4.8)$$

Two multislice loop structures are commonly used. Traditional multislice looping uses $N_{\text{SUBLOOP}} = 1$ (Figure 4.10a), so that one line of data is acquired for each slice prior to measurement of a second line of data from any slice. The maximum number of slices is limited by *TR*. This provides the most efficient data collection process for a given *TR* and is useful when *TR* is relatively long. At the midpoint of a scan using this looping scheme, each image has $N_{\text{PE}}/2$ lines of raw data, each with the requested number of acquisitions.

The other approach uses N_{SUBLOOP} equal to the number of slices (Figure 4.10b), a so-called sequential slice technique. In this technique, all information for a slice is acquired before acquiring any information for another slice. Only one line of data is measured during each *TR* time period. This allows the use of very short *TR* times when acquiring large numbers of slices. At the midpoint of a scan using this looping scheme, all the data for one-half the requested number of slices has been acquired.

There is also variability in the order of the main loops for 2D multislice imaging. Traditional looping as in Figure 4.10a acquires all signals for a specified phase encoding step (all slices, all averages) before acquiring a signal for a different phase encoding step. This allows all signal averaging for a given raw data line to be done within a short period of time and allows initial steps of image reconstruction to be performed. The other variation acquires a complete raw data set

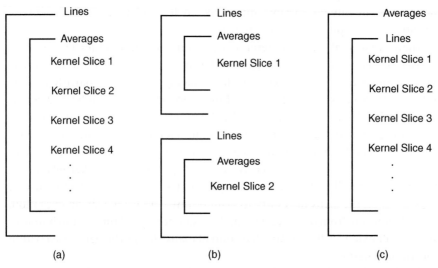

Figure 4.10 Two-dimensional slice loop structures. Three slice loop structures are commonly used. (a) Traditional multislice looping. The slice loop is the innermost loop ($N_{\text{SUBLOOP}} = 1$ not indicated). Each slice is excited and signal-detected prior to any slice being excited a second time for purposes of signal averaging or phase encoding (lines). This loop structure is the most common. (b) Sequential slice looping. All information for a given slice is acquired prior to any excitation for a different slice. In this figure, $N_{\text{SUBLOOP}} = 2$. (c) Long-term averaging. All lines for all slices are acquired before performing signal averaging.

for a slice before beginning any signal averaging (Figure 4.10c). This increases the elapsed time between successive signals being averaged together, reducing any possible contamination between the signals, but renders the image more susceptible to gross patient motion.

The other category of measurement technique is a 3D volume acquisition, which is, in essence, a double phase encoding technique. For 3D volume imaging, tissue volumes of 30–150 mm are excited as compared to 3–10 mm in 2D imaging. In addition, a second phase encoding table is applied in the slice selection direction to "partition" or subdivide the volume into individual slices. Each echo is acquired following application of encoding gradients in both the phase encoding and slice selection directions, one amplitude from each.

The advantages of 3D volume acquisition techniques are that the slices within a volume are contiguous and that the detected signal is based on the total volume of excitation rather than the effective slice thickness. The 3D volume acquisitions have two primary disadvantages. Because of the potentially long scan times, they are usually gradient echo or echo train spin echo sequences and are limited to one or two volumes. Image processing is also longer since an additional Fourier transformation and other processing steps must be performed in order to produce an image.

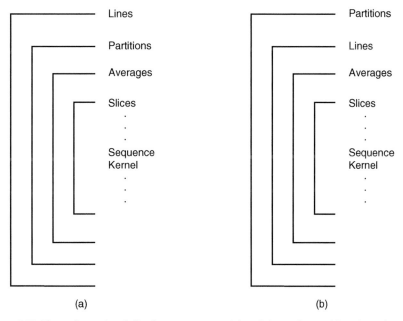

Figure 4.11 Three-dimensional slice loop structures. A fourth loop, the partitions loop, is added. Two slice loop structures are commonly used: (a) partitions-in-lines: the partitions gradient amplitudes are varied most frequently; (b) lines-in-partitions: the lines gradient amplitudes are varied most frequently.

For 3D volume MRI techniques, in each excitation volume the number of slices is determined by the number of partitions, N_{PART}. The total scan time is:

$$(\text{Scan time})_{3D} = TR * N_{SA} * N_{PE} * N_{PART} * N_{SUBLOOP} \tag{4.9}$$

There are two possibilities for the order of the two encoding loops. Traditional looping has the partitions loop inside the phase encoding loop (Figure 4.11a), typical of 3D gradient echo techniques. Since the partitions loop normally has fewer entries, this enables initial image processing to be performed while data collection continues. The other order has the phase encoding loop inside the partitions loop (Figure 4.11b). This is more typical for 3D echo train spin echo, where the phase encoding loop is segmented in nature (see Chapter 5).

CHAPTER 5

Principles of magnetic resonance imaging – 2

The basic steps for spatial localization of the MR signal were described in Chapter 4. These steps (slice selection, frequency and phase encoding, looping) are common features of nearly all MRI measurements. While the descriptions in Chapter 4 are generally correct as presented, there are additional concepts that are integral to the process and must be considered in order to obtain an accurate understanding of MRI. In most cases, the concepts presented here may be implemented with any of the MRI measurement techniques described in the next chapter.

5.1 Frequency selective excitation

Chapter 2 presented the general concepts of RF excitation and resonance absorption by the protons. The nature of the RF transmitter is described in more detail in Chapter 14, but its basic nature is to amplify or increase the amplitude of an input waveform. MRI scanners manipulate the input RF waveforms via software to achieve the desired output of the transmitter. In principle, the RF transmitter can operate in one of two modes: continuous wave and pulse. Continuous wave (CW) mode operation broadcasts the RF energy at all times. Due to its demands on the transmitter hardware, the output power and frequency range are typically limited. While used in MR scanners historically, CW mode is seldom used in MRI scanners today and will not be discussed further in this book. Pulsed mode operation broadcasts energy for brief periods of time and is the standard operational mode for MRI scanners. The peak power produced by the transmitter is greater than with CW operation, but a wider range of frequencies can be manipulated with greater precision. This increased flexibility is achieved through shaping or crafting the pulse prior to amplification to obtain the desired output.

The RF waveform consists of a set of complex data points with amplitudes and phases that vary with time, typically several hundred in number. These digital points are converted to analog format prior to mixing with the base

MRI Basic Principles and Applications, Fifth Edition.
Brian M. Dale, Mark A. Brown and Richard C. Semelka.
© 2015 John Wiley & Sons, Ltd. Published 2015 by John Wiley & Sons, Ltd.

or carrier frequency and amplification. There are several parameters that are used to characterize RF waveforms. Depending on the manufacturer's software, some of these parameters may be accessible to the operator while others may be predefined:

Center frequency. The center frequency of the pulse is normally chosen as the resonant frequency for the particular collection of protons to be excited. For example, this may be a slice for slice selection or spatial presaturation, or fat protons for fat saturation.

Duration. The pulse duration is the length of time that the waveform is broadcast. It is inversely proportional to the bandwidth or range of frequencies that are broadcast by the transmitter; narrower bandwidth pulses require longer RF pulse durations.

Phase. The phase of the pulse defines the effective orientation of the RF energy (see Figure 2.2) and determines the axis of rotation for the net magnetization under the influence of the pulse.

Amplitude. The pulse amplitude, or, more precisely, the pulse amplitude integral, determines the amount of rotation that the protons undergo (flip angle). In addition, the pulse amplitude is related to the amount of energy (power) that the protons absorb and therefore must dissipate through $T1$ relaxation.

Nature of synthesizer mixing (modulation). More details of the combination of the RF waveform with the frequency synthesizer are described in Chapter 14. As mentioned previously, the RF pulse waveforms contain a range of frequencies that will be excited by the pulse. There are two methods that are used for merging the waveform with the center frequency produced by the frequency synthesizer:

- Amplitude modulation distributes the energy to all frequencies at the same time during the pulse. This mode ensures that all frequencies are treated equally by the RF transmitter.
- Frequency/phase modulation excites each frequency/phase sequentially during application of the pulse, each at the same amplitude. These pulses frequently are less demanding on the transmitter hardware in terms of peak power output, but require more total power from the transmitter.

Regardless of the type of modulation, most MRI applications require uniform behavior of the frequencies encompassed by the RF pulse by the end of transmission; that is, the RF pulse excites all frequencies equally within its selected range. This translates into a pulse waveform that produces uniform amplitude and phase excitation throughout the frequency range; that is, all affected protons should be rotated the same amount and in the same direction when the transmitter is turned off. This ensures that all protons within the excitation volume will have a common starting point following the excitation process.

Pulse shape. The pulse shape is the mathematical function that best models the waveform in time (the time-domain shape is used as this is the format used as input to the transmitter). There are four shapes that are frequently used:

- *Nonselective* pulses, also known as rectangular or "hard" pulses, are of short duration and constant amplitude and excite a broad frequency range with a uniform amplitude. They are usually used to determine the resonant frequency of the patient or if very short RF pulse durations are required. Nonselective pulses may also be used in a series of pulses applied in a very short time period, known as a composite pulse (see Section 5.2). Strictly speaking, "nonselective" pulses are frequency selective since the pulsed nature of the excitation limits the frequency bandwidth that can be incorporated into the pulse (Figure 5.1).

    The remaining pulses are collectively known as frequency selective or "soft" pulses. Frequency-selective pulses do not have a constant amplitude at all times or at all frequencies during broadcasting. Their pulse durations are longer than for a nonselective pulse, allowing for a narrower frequency bandwidth; however, they are still truncated or shortened in time compared to the theoretical pulse shapes, which have infinitely long durations:

- *Sinc* pulses are the primary choice as frequency-selective excitation and refocusing pulses. These pulses provide uniform amplitude and phase excitation throughout the slice. For an RF pulse to excite a particular frequency, that frequency must be included within its bandwidth. As more frequencies at the same phase are included in a pulse, the pulse shape approaches that of a sinc function, an infinite function that contains all possible frequencies in the bandwidth (Figure 5.2). Due to the short duration of the pulse

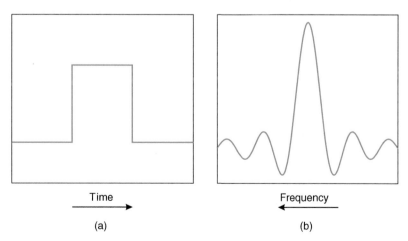

Time →

Frequency ←

(a)   (b)

Figure 5.1 Nonselective or rectangular RF pulse: (a) time-domain waveform; (b) frequency-domain waveform.

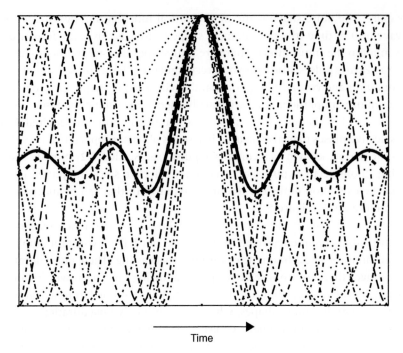

Time

Figure 5.2 A series of sine waves of different frequencies all in phase at one point in time sum to give an approximation (dashed dark line) of an infinite sinc function (solid dark line).

and its limited bandwidth, the actual pulse shape used for slice selective pulses is a truncated sinc function. This truncation causes the frequency cutoff to be less than ideal, with two important consequences: frequencies outside the desired bandwidth are excited as well as those within the bandwidth and the drop-off of the excitation (known as the pulse profile) is not rectangular but has sloped sides. The extraneous excitation can be minimized by filtering the sinc function or mathematically forcing it to zero at the edges. This reduces the total power contained within the pulse, but accentuates the sloped nature of the pulse profile (Figure 5.3).

- *Gaussian* pulses are frequently used for frequency-selective saturation pulses such as fat suppression or magnetization transfer suppression due to a narrower excitation bandwidth (see Chapter 7). These pulses have excitation profiles that follow a Gaussian shape, which is more rounded than the sinc function (Figure 5.4). These pulses are also frequently filtered, which affects the frequency bandwidth.
- *Hyperbolic secant* pulses are often used as inversion pulses in inversion recovery sequences (see Chapter 6). These pulses are applied as phase-modulated adiabatic (literally, "no heat") pulses and produce inversion of the net magnetization with very uniform frequency profiles independent of transmitter amplitude levels. Hyperbolic secant pulses have phase variations that make them unsuitable for use as a refocusing pulse (Figure 5.5). They also generally have higher power deposition that either sinc or Gaussian pulses.

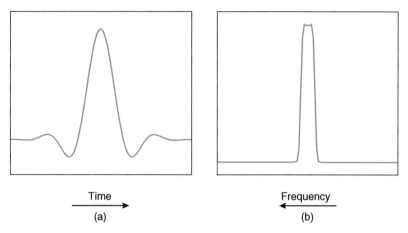

Figure 5.3 Truncated sinc RF pulse: (a) time-domain waveform; (b) frequency-domain waveform.

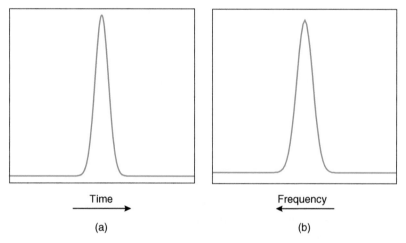

Figure 5.4 Gaussian RF pulse: (a) time-domain waveform; (b) frequency-domain waveform.

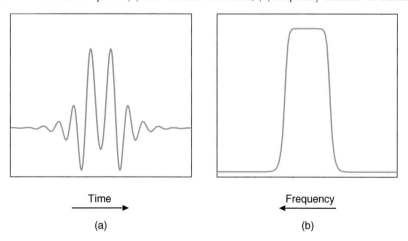

Figure 5.5 Hyperbolic secant or adiabatic RF pulse: (a) time-domain waveform; (b) frequency-domain waveform.

In general, RF excitation pulses are subject to several competing criteria:

1 Short duration pulses require high peak pulse amplitudes to achieve the same pulse area (flip angle). Depending on the particular RF amplifier and transmitter coil, the maximum power that can be broadcast is limited.

2 As the pulse amplitude increases, the power deposited by the pulse also increases in a quadratic fashion (a factor of two increase in the pulse amplitude causes a factor of four in the pulse power). This fact may require longer pulse durations to minimize RF power deposition, which may require an increase in *TE* and *TR*.

3 Sinc functions produce rectangular, phase coherent excitation profiles only with low flip angles (<30°). High amplitude sinc pulses such as 90° or 180° pulses have excitation profiles that are significantly nonrectangular. Manufacturers strive to provide uniform excitation profiles, subject to the other criteria. Specific questions about particular RF pulse profiles should be addressed to the individual manufacturer.

4 As the RF pulse duration increases, the bandwidth of the pulse decreases. This means that less G_{SS} is required to focus the energy to the same tissue volume. However, as G_{SS} is reduced, the sharpness of the slice profile (known as the transition region) is reduced as well. This can cause more pronounced crosstalk between slices or sensitivity to magnetic susceptibility differences within the slice, producing nonuniform image intensities, particularly at ultra-high field strengths.

5.2 Composite pulses

The RF pulses described above are typically applied as a single unit; that is, the manipulations of the spin are performed by a single waveform that is broadcast at the appropriate time. A composite RF pulse is a series of closely spaced RF pulses applied over a short time period that together affect the protons like a single pulse. The pulse amplitudes for each RF pulse typically form a binomial progression (e.g., 11, 121, 1331), with the effective flip angle being the sum of the individual flip angles. The timing between the pulses allows protons with different resonant frequencies to cycle in phase and undergo different effects from each pulse (Figure 5.6). The individual pulses may be nonselective (rectangular) or frequency selective, resulting in a composite pulse of the same character. In general, composite pulses require less transmitter power than single RF pulses for the same flip angle because of the short duration of the individual pulses. However, the total time required for the combined excitation is longer than for a single excitation pulse. Composite pulses can be used for general slice excitation, but the most common application is for signal suppression (see Chapter 8).

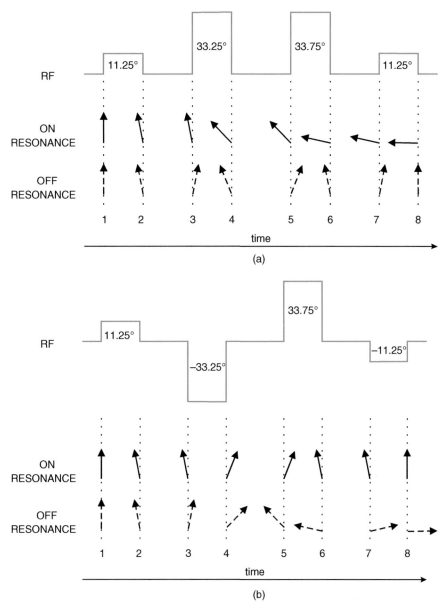

Figure 5.6 Composite pulses. (a) A 1331 composite pulse is shown with a total excitation angle of 90°. A rotating frame corresponding to the on-resonant frequency is assumed. Prior to the first RF pulse (1), both on-resonance (solid arrow) and off-resonance (dashed arrow) protons are unexcited. At the end of the first RF pulse (2), both will be excited 11.25°. Because of the difference in resonant frequencies, the off-resonance protons become out of phase. The time for the second RF pulse (3) is chosen so that the off-resonance protons are exactly 180° out of phase. At the end of the second RF pulse (4), the on-resonance protons are excited 45° while the on-resonance protons are excited 22.5°. The delay between the second and third RF pulses is chosen so that the off-resonance protons are 180° out of phase with the on-resonance proton (5). A similar delay is chosen between the third and fourth RF pulses (6,7). At the end of the fourth RF pulse (8), the on-resonance protons are rotated 90° (excited), while the off-resonance protons are at 0° (unexcited). (b) A 1331 composite pulse with a total excitation angle of 90°. The end result differs from (a) in that the on-resonance spins are not excited while the off-resonance spins are rotated 90°.

5.3 Raw data and image data matrices

 In analyzing measured MRI data, two formats for the data may be used: raw data and image data. Both data sets contain the same information from the slice or slices and both formats are used for different purposes. They are stored and manipulated as a grid or matrix of points representing the slice. The two formats are related by the Fourier transformation, with the raw data being the format generated by and used in the data collection process and the image data being the format normally used for viewing and interpretation.

In MRI, the raw data consists of the digitized data measured for a given echo from a given slice or volume of tissue. Whether an analog or digital receiver is used (see Chapter 14), the echo signal amplitude measured by the receiver coil is digitized as a function of time. The amplitude variations have a shape roughly corresponding to a sinc function (see Figure 5.2). The digital form of the signal is stored as a complex data array with each signal point represented by real and imaginary values. For the raw data matrix, the detected signal amplitudes for a given echo correspond to a row and each row differs by the value of G_{PE} applied prior to detection. The rows are typically displayed in order of increasing phase encoding amplitudes from top to bottom, corresponding to maximum negative to maximum positive G_{PE} amplitudes, respectively. The raw data matrix is thus a grid of points with the readout direction displayed in the horizontal direction and the phase encoding direction displayed in the vertical direction. Its dimensions depend on the number of readout data points and the number of phase encoding steps for the scan (Figure 5.7).

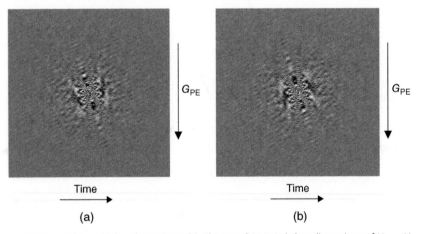

Figure 5.7 Raw data, real (a) and imaginary (b). The raw data matrix has dimensions of $N_{PE} \times N_{RO}$. Each row is a measured signal at a particular G_{PE}. The number of rows corresponds to N_{PE}. Signals acquired with high negative amplitude G_{PE} are displayed at the top, low amplitude G_{PE} in the middle, and high positive amplitude G_{PE} at the bottom of the matrix. Each column corresponds to a data point sampled at a different time following the excitation pulse.

The image data or display matrix is obtained via the 2D Fourier transformation (rows and columns) of the complex raw data matrix. The image matrix is a

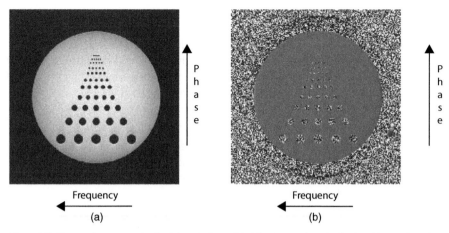

Figure 5.8 Image data, magnitude (a) and phase (b). The image data is obtained by performing a two-dimensional Fourier transformation on the data set displayed in Figure 5.7. The rows and columns correspond to the phase-encoding and readout directions. The specification of rows and columns as readout and phase-encoding directions is usually set by the operator.

complex frequency and phase map of the proton signal intensity from a volume element weighted by the *T1* and *T2* values of the tissues contained within the volume. The specific frequencies and phases are unique to the location of the volume element and are measured relative to the base transmitter frequency. Rather than viewing images as complex arrays, the displayed image matrix is normally an array of real or integer values, consisting either of the signal magnitudes or the relative phases at each point. Although they must be the same dimension as the raw data matrix, image matrices are usually displayed as square arrays with readout as one direction and phase encoding as the other direction in the image (Figure 5.8). To accomplish this, a process known as interpolation may be performed in which additional image pixels are created by the Fourier transformation process that are derived from the original pixels. For example, if a 192 PE × 256 RO matrix is acquired, the image that results is 256 rows × 256 columns, with 64 "extra" pixels created in the PE direction by the Fourier transformation. The choice of rows and columns for readout and phase encoding is at the operator's discretion and is normally made to minimize artifacts in the area of interest. The maximum dimensions in the displayed image matrix normally correspond to the chosen FOV in each direction.

5.4 Signal-to-noise ratio and tradeoffs

 One of the most important characteristics of both the raw data and image data is the signal-to-noise ratio (SNR). The SNR of MRI data depends on both the level of signal and the level of noise present in the data, each of which depends on many factors. A voxel with a larger volume contains more signal, and therefore has a higher SNR. Longer sampling time reduces the noise, and therefore increases the SNR. In addition, the MRI hardware contributes to the SNR through the main magnetic field strength, the receive coil sensitivity and volume, and the receive chain noise performance characteristics. Finally, the tissue itself contributes to the signal as determined by its relaxation and other characteristics that affect the specific pulse sequence being used. These effects can be stated as follows:

$$SNR = V * T^{1/2} * R(B0, B1, \ldots) * I_{seq}(T1, T2, TE, TR, \ldots) \qquad (5.1)$$

where V is the voxel volume, T is the total sampling time for each voxel, R is a factor characterizing the SNR of the hardware and processing chain including the main magnetic field, the receive coil sensitivity, and so forth, and I_{seq} is a factor characterizing the signal intensity from the pulse sequence and the tissue.

In equation (5.1) the factor R is generally considered fixed since alterations to R usually require the purchase of a new MRI system or new MRI receive coils. Similarly, I_{seq} is fixed in the sense that it contains the information that is desired from the MRI exam. It is the interaction of the pulse sequence with the tissue that emphasizes the tissue characteristics in the measured signal, so changes to I_{seq} would change the diagnostic information in the image.

 This leaves V and T as the only free parameters that can be varied as needed for a given patient in order to improve SNR. Equation (5.1) shows that the SNR is proportional to the voxel volume and the square root of the sampling time. This represents the fundamental compromise, or tradeoff, of MR imaging. If an improvement in the SNR is required, then either spatial resolution or sampling time must be sacrificed. If an improvement in spatial resolution is required, then either SNR will be reduced or sampling time will be increased, etc.

5.5 Raw data and *k*-space

The raw data matrix is a significant concept in MRI. Prior to data processing, each slice will be represented by a raw data matrix. All the information necessary to reconstruct an image is contained within the raw data matrix. Each data point contributes to all aspects (frequency, phase, and amplitude) of every location within the slice, though some data points emphasize different features in the final image. The maximum signal content is located in the central portion of the raw data matrix. These lines are acquired with low amplitude G_{PE} and the measured signal amplitude variations are predominantly due to differences in the inherent tissue signals. These lines are primarily responsible for the contrast in the image. The outer portions of the raw data matrix have relatively low signal amplitude and are acquired with either high positive amplitude or high negative

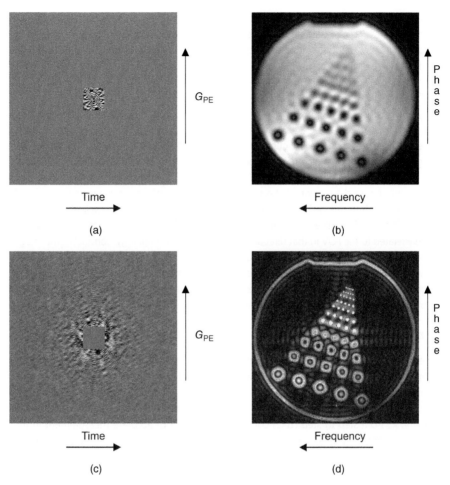

Figure 5.9 Raw data and corresponding images. (a) Same raw data set as Figure 5.7 except that only the central 32 × 32 data points are kept and zero values are defined for the remaining data. Imaginary portion not shown. (b) Magnitude image data of (a). The image intensity is approximately the same as that of Figure 5.8a, but there is a loss of edge definition, exhibited as blurring in the phantom. (c) Same raw data set as Figure 5.7 except that the central 32 × 32 data points are eliminated, corresponding to 1.56% of the total data set. Imaginary portion not shown. (d) Magnitude image data of (c). The image intensity (central portion of the phantom) is virtually absent, while the edges of the phantom are present.

amplitude G_{PE}. These gradients produce high frequencies (by the Larmor equation) and provide mainly edge definition to the resultant image (Figure 5.9).

An alternate method to describe the raw data matrix is called the k-space formalism. It provides a convenient way to describe methods for acquiring raw data. In this approach, the complex array of raw data points is treated as a two-dimensional grid of points (k_x, k_y). Each k_x value corresponds to a point in the readout direction of the raw data matrix and each k_y value corresponds to a point in the phase encoding direction of the raw data matrix. Each (k_x, k_y) data point corresponds to the echo signal amplitude influenced by the combination of readout and phase encoding gradient areas or moments (time * gradient amplitude):

$$k_x = \gamma G_{RO} t_{RO}$$

$$k_y = \gamma G_{PE} t_{PE} \tag{5.2}$$

where t_{RO}, t_{PE} corresponds to the cumulative time that the respective gradient is active. The total gradient influence at each (k_x, k_y) point in the matrix is different and unique. The point (0, 0), referred to as the origin of k-space, has the maximum amplitude in the raw data matrix ($G_{PE} = 0$, maximum data point of the echo signal). The k values are measured in units of mm^{-1} and are often referred to as spatial frequencies, in analogy with cyclical frequencies measured in units of s^{-1}. The change in k in each direction from point to point (Δk_x or Δk_y) is inversely related to the FOV in that direction. Using k-space terminology, contrast in the image is primarily determined by low spatial frequency data near the center while edge definition is primarily determined by high spatial frequency data at the edges of k-space.

For 3D volume scanning, the k-space description requires the addition of a third dimension, k_z, corresponding to the partitions gradient mentioned in Chapter 4:

$$k_z = \gamma G_{SS} t_{SS} \tag{5.3}$$

where t_{SS} is the cumulative time that the slice selection gradient G_{SS} is active. In general, the principles discussed above for k-space of two-dimensional images are also true for 3D volume scanning. The raw data space is a three-dimensional volume defined with three coordinates (k_x, k_y, k_z), analogous to the two-dimensional volume defined by (k_x, k_y) described earlier. The change in k_z from step to step (Δk_z) controls the distance of accurate measurement in the slice direction (typically matching the volume of RF excitation). The origin of the volume (0, 0, 0) contributes most to the contrast and the edges of the k volume contribute edge definition in the resulting images. The 3D looping structures illustrated in Figure 4.11 can be identified as the two ordering schemes for varying the k_y and k_z gradient amplitudes, either fixed k_z-varying k_y or fixed k_y-varying k_z, respectively.

Two requirements to produce artifact-free images are for the raw data space to be sampled continuously (no gaps in lines or columns) and with a uniform density in a given direction. In terms of k-space, Δk_x and Δk_y must be constant but not necessarily equal and must span the entire space. This requirement ensures equal weight to both contrast and edge definition in the final image. One approach to accomplish these requirements, used in traditional scanning, involves a rectilinear data collection. Each MR signal is measured in the presence of a constant amplitude G_{RO} with the same number of sample points measured at a constant rate (constant dwell time). The phase encoding gradient G_{PE} is changed by a constant increment (ΔG_{PE}) from line to line (Figure 5.10). When a complete set of G_{PE} lines is acquired, a raw data set is produced that fulfills both criteria.

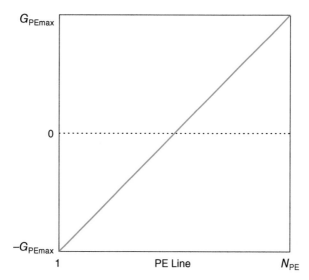

Figure 5.10 Sequential k-space filling. Each line of k-space (phase-encoding line) corresponds to a measured MR signal. Lines of k-space are acquired serially in time with the data from the maximum negative G_{PE} acquired first and the data from the maximum positive G_{PE} acquired last. The center of k-space ($G_{PE} = 0$ mT m^{-1}) step is acquired halfway through the data collection period. This is the traditional data collection method.

5.6 Reduced *k*-space techniques

The requirements for continuity and uniform density of the raw data matrix do not require that a complete raw data be measured in order to produce artifact-free images. Since many MRI scans are several minutes in duration, methods to reduce the scan time while maintaining image fidelity are desirable. Since the scan time is proportional to the number of phase encoding steps N_{PE}, a common approach to reduce the scan time is to reduce the number of measured G_{PE} amplitudes. If the measured amplitudes are properly chosen, then the above-mentioned requirements can be fulfilled. Two approaches reduce the total number of G_{PE} amplitudes symmetrically around $G_{PE} = 0$. One method keeps the change in amplitude ΔG_{PE} between successive steps (or, equivalently, Δk_y) equal to that for the "complete" raw data matrix, so that the FOV in the phase encoding direction is the same in both images. The maximum G_{PE} values are smaller than those for the complete raw data matrix. The missing lines are replaced by zeros prior to Fourier transformation, a process known as zero-filling, so that the final image matrix is square, as described in Section 5.2. This results in a loss of spatial resolution in the final image due to the loss of information at high spatial frequencies (Figure 5.11). The other method increases ΔG_{PE} (Δk_y) so that the maximum G_{PE} values are equal to the complete raw data matrix. In this case, the FOV in the phase encoding direction is reduced, regaining the loss in spatial resolution due to the reduced number of lines. However, the spatial region of accurate phase measurement is reduced, potentially causing aliasing artifacts. These may be detrimental to the image quality (see Chapter 9) or used

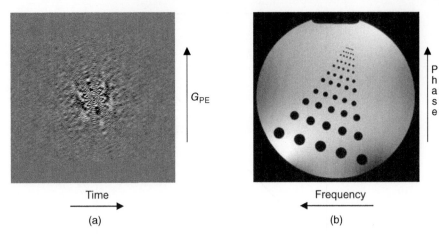

Time G_{PE} Frequency   Phase

(a)   (b)

Figure 5.11 Raw data and corresponding image. (a) Raw data set for 192 lines measured with the same ΔG_{PE} as for Figure 5.7, and zero values are defined for the remaining data. Imaginary portion not shown. (b) Magnitude image data of (a). The FOV is identical and the image intensity is almost identical to that of Figure 5.8a, but there is a slight loss of edge definition, exhibited as blurring in the phantom.

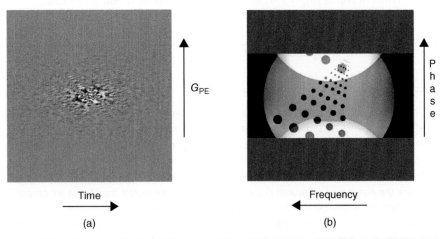

Time G_{PE} Frequency   Phase

(a)   (b)

Figure 5.12 Raw data and corresponding image. (a) Raw data set for 192 lines measured with an increased ΔG_{PE} compared to Figure 5.7, and zero values are defined for the remaining data. Imaginary portion not shown. (b) Magnitude image data of (a). The FOV is reduced compared to that of Figure 5.8a, causing aliasing artifact. (a) (b) GPE

as part of the data collection process (see Section 5.10). In addition, the final image is often padded with extra lines to make the final image display square, which reduces the portion of the total image that contains useful information (Figure 5.12). Use of a reduced number of G_{PE} lines (e.g., 192 PE lines × 256 RO points) also fulfills the requirement for a "continuous" k-space, since the "missing" lines are at the edges of k-space and that there are no gaps in the interior.

A third method for reducing the number of measured raw data lines is known as partial Fourier imaging. Due to the usage of positive and negative polarity G_{PE} gradients, a symmetry to the raw data matrix is generated. This symmetry is known as Hermitian symmetry, with the negative amplitude gradients producing real signals with the same amplitude and opposite phases as the signals generated by the positive amplitude gradients (Figure 5.13). The partial Fourier technique reduces the total number of lines acquired for the raw data matrix, but in an asymmetric fashion about the $G_{PE} = 0$ line. The maximum amplitude G_{PE} and ΔG_{PE} between each acquisition are the same as for a complete raw data matrix, maintaining the spatial resolution and FOV, respectively. The missing raw data (high positive amplitude G_{PE}) are extrapolated from the measured data through the Hermitian symmetry prior to Fourier transformation. The resulting image has the same FOV and spatial resolution as that from a complete raw data matrix, but the scan time is reduced. The problems with partial Fourier techniques are a loss in SNR due to the reduced number of measured lines (reduced T in equation (5.1)) and an enhanced sensitivity to artifacts due to the artificial replication of the information; in effect, an artifactual signal is duplicated rather than being averaged.

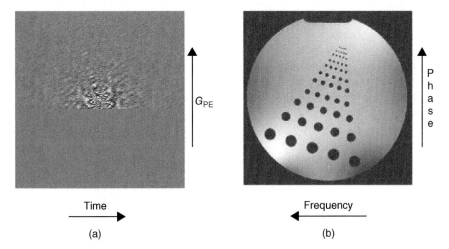

Figure 5.13 Raw data and corresponding image. (a) Same raw data set as Figure 5.7 except that only the upper 136 lines are kept, and zero values are defined for the remaining data. Imaginary portion not shown. (b) Magnitude image data of (a). The spatial resolution and signal intensity are identical to those of Figure 5.8a, but there is a slight increase in noise.

Reduction of data in the readout direction is also possible; however, the scan time is not directly affected. These methods typically involve reducing the number of sample points for the echo while maintaining G_{RO} and the dwell time. This allows a shorter total sampling time to be used, reducing the sequence kernel time and allowing a shorter minimum TR to be used or more slices to be measured. This reduced sampling can be performed symmetrically with zero-filling or, asymmetrically, producing a half-echo. In this case, as in the case of a partial Fourier in the PE direction, the missing data are extrapolated based on the Hermitian symmetry of the echo.

5.7 Reordered *k*-space filling techniques

While a complete *k*-space of uniform density is necessary prior to Fourier transformation, the order in which the individual k_y lines are acquired is somewhat arbitrary. This filling order is also known as the *k*-space trajectory. The traditional method for data collection is sequential filling or a linear trajectory. The raw data matrix is filled, one line at a time, with adjacent k_y lines acquired serially in time. The readout gradient G_{RO} is applied for a constant period of time and amplitude, during which time the echo is sampled with a constant dwell time. Depending on the particular manufacturer and pulse sequence, the scan may begin with the most negative G_{PE} and end with the most positive G_{PE} (increasing amplitudes) or the opposite (decreasing amplitudes). In either case, G_{PE} is varied in a linear fashion and the $k_y = 0$ signal is measured halfway through the data collection (see Figure 5.10).

Other methods for filling *k*-space are used for special applications or when additional contrast control is required. Reordered *k*-space refers to methods of data collection where the raw data are acquired in a nonsequential fashion. Centric ordering acquires the low amplitude G_{PE} steps earliest in the scan, with higher amplitude G_{PE} steps acquired later (Figure 5.14). Variations on sequential and centric ordering are possible, in which the $k_y = 0$ signal is acquired at other times of the scan. These approaches may be useful in scans where the net magnetization **M** is not sufficiently close to a steady-state value in the initial detected echoes. Acquiring the $k_y = 0$ signal at a time shortly after the scan begins will allow **M** to reach a value closer to the steady-state value using the initial RF excitation pulses of the sequence rather than "dummy" excitation pulses.

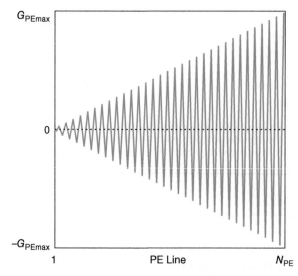

Figure 5.14 Centric *k*-space filling. Lines of *k*-space are acquired serially beginning at the center of *k*-space, then in increasing G_{PE} amplitudes of alternating polarity.

Another useful approach for data collection is the segmented method, in which successive echoes in the scan measure lines from different regions or segments of k-space. Data are collected in a segment-serial fashion, one phase encoding step from each segment. The number of segments, the number of lines per segment, and the order of acquisition may be independently varied (Figure 5.15), though the total number of measured lines will be the product of the number of lines per segment times the number of segments.

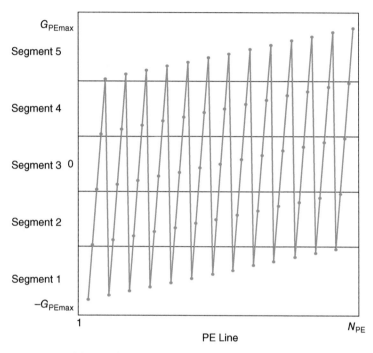

Figure 5.15 Segmented k-space filling. Lines of k-space are acquired in groups or segments. The example here shows five segments. One line of data is acquired from each segment before a second line is acquired from any segment. The center of k-space is acquired at a time during the scan that is dependent on the number of lines per segment, number of segments, and the order of acquisition within a segment and between segments.

For 3D scanning, the reordering of k-space can be done in different ways. The two gradient tables (k_y and k_z) are independent of each other and need not be varied in the same fashion. For example, one table may be sequential stepping while the other may be centric or segmented. Spiral scanning in 3D refers to the stepping order of the $k_y - k_z$ gradients in which the two amplitude variations form a spiral (Figure 5.16). This approach is useful in acquiring the contrast-determining echoes early in the measurement, allowing control of tissue contrast, or minimizing motion artifacts.

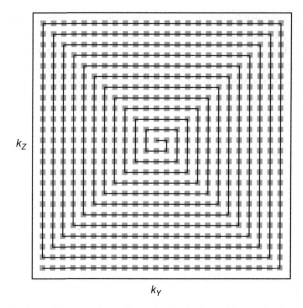

k_Z

k_Y

Figure 5.16 Spiral filling of k-space, three-dimensional. The k_y and k_z amplitudes are varied in an increasing spiral pattern. The lowest-amplitude values are used to acquire the earliest echoes in the scan.

5.8 Other k-space filling techniques

As mentioned in Section 5.3, a continuous (gap-free) raw data set of uniform density must be acquired prior to Fourier transformation to minimize image artifacts. This may be accomplished in several ways. Conventional scan techniques sample the echo signal with a constant dwell time and a constant G_{RO} and use a G_{PE} that varies with constant increment. This is the easiest approach to ensure a constant Δk_x and Δk_y. Nonrectilinear sampling occurs when either of these conditions is not fulfilled. Three important examples of this are ramped sampling, spiral sampling, and radial sampling.

Ramped sampling is a simple variation from the traditional rectilinear sampling. A normal gradient pulse consists of two amplitude-varying parts known as the ramps (a ramp up and a ramp down) and a constant amplitude portion known as the plateau or flat-top (see Chapter 6). If sampling of the echo occurs while G_{RO} is changing (sampling during the ramp time), the effect of G_{RO} will not be uniform for each sample point of the echo (Δk_x will not be constant) (Figure 5.17). Ramped sampling may be desired in order to obtain specific measurement parameters (for instance, a shorter TE). The problem of variable Δk_x when performing ramped sampling can be eliminated either by using variable dwell time sampling, ensuring that Δk_x is constant during sampling, or by

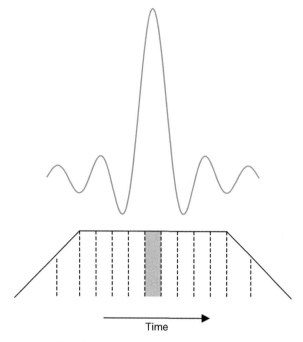

Time

Figure 5.17 Ramped sampling of signal. The dashed lines represent the time points when signal sampling occurs. The G_{RO} gradient amplitude is not constant during signal sampling. As a result, Δk_x, which is proportional to the rectangular gray area, is not constant for all sample points.

performing a regridding of the measured data prior to Fourier transformation. Regridding creates a constant Δk_x from the measured data using interpolation methods to generate the missing data points. The computational difficulty of the regridding method depends on the nature of the G_{RO} variation. Ramped sampling is similar to conventional sampling in that the readout process (G_{RO} and sampling rate) are identical for all echoes used to generate the image.

The other approaches have G_{RO} values that differ from echo to echo. One method is known as projection reconstruction, frequently implemented as radial scanning. Projection reconstruction uses a constant G_{RO} but its direction changes from echo to echo. The two gradients that are perpendicular to G_{SS} are combined with different ratios, which generate different perspectives or projections of the slice. Each digitized signal produces a line of raw data, but the lines are in different directions (Figure 5.18). One advantage of radial scanning is that each echo samples the center of k-space, so that each signal will have an equivalent SNR. The primary disadvantage is that the sampling density of k-space will not be uniform (the points near the center of k-space (Δk_x, $\Delta k_y \approx 0$) are sampled more densely than those near the edges of k-space). Also, Δk_x and Δk_y will normally not be constant. As a result, a regridding of the raw data must be performed prior to Fourier transformation in order to produce images without phase artifacts. In addition,

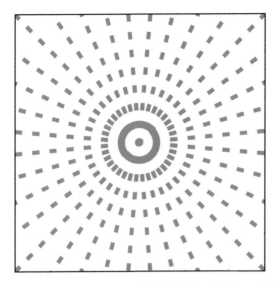

Figure 5.18 Radial filling of k-space. Each signal is sampled with a $\boldsymbol{G_{RO}}$ gradient consisting of the sum of two physical gradients with variable amplitudes. The direction of each $\boldsymbol{G_{RO}}$ varies depending on the particular gradient amplitudes.

all echoes will contribute significantly to the image contrast. Any hardware imperfections or patient motion at any point in the scan will produce artifacts.

While radial scanning uses varying G_{RO}, its magnitude is constant during each line. Two-dimensional spiral sampling is a technique where the G_{RO} gradient amplitude varies in magnitude during the echo sampling. Specifically, the two gradients perpendicular to G_{SS} are both varied in a spiral fashion during the echo sampling. This has the result of generating a raw dataset that has data points forming a spiral k-space (Figure 5.19). The central points of k-space are usually acquired early in the data collection period, as this allows a shorter *TE* to be used. Regridding in both k_x and k_y is necessary to ensure a constant density k-space prior to Fourier transformation.

5.9 Phased-array coils

In Chapter 2, the use of a receiver coil in the MR measurement process was described. Receiver coils have many different sizes and shapes, but have one common characteristic: their effective axis (or coil axis) is always normal or per-pendicular to $\boldsymbol{B_0}$. For loop coils (consisting of a loop of wire), the effective axis is normal to the direction of the loop. For other coil designs, the effective axis is less obvious, but will always be perpendicular to $\boldsymbol{B_0}$ in all cases.

Another consideration in coil design is the sensitive volume for the coil. For simple loop-type coils, the sensitive volume is roughly equal to one radius in

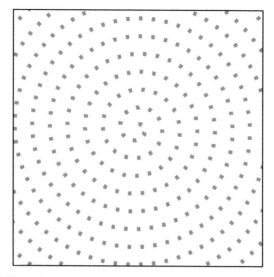

Figure 5.19 Spiral filling of k-space, two-dimensional. The signal is sampled with the gradients perpendicular to G_{SS} varying in a spiral fashion.

distance normal to the surface of the coil; in other words, the coil penetration is approximately one radius in distance from the surface of the loop. One type of coil, known as a surface coil, consists of one or more loops. These coils are most sensitive to signals from tissue near the surface of the coil with progressively less signal from tissue farther away from the coil surface. The size of the loop is a significant factor in the coil sensitivity, with larger coils being less sensitive. This is caused by a property known as the coil loading (see Chapter 14), in which the patient coupling or loading of the coil affects the coil sensitivity. It is important that the patient anatomy fill the coil-sensitive volume as much as possible to ensure that the coil operates most efficiently.

For surface coils such as those used for spine imaging, this loss of sensitivity limits the size of the coil that can be used effectively, and the associated anatomical coverage. To overcome this limitation, multiple smaller coils known as phased-array coils have been developed. These coils are arranged in such a manner that they do not interfere with each other (little mutual inductance). Each individual coil in the array is an independent receiver coil that measures the signal from its sensitive area (Figure 5.20). A complete k-space is acquired and processed for each coil in the array. The resulting "subimages" are combined to produce an image from a larger anatomical region than is possible for an individual coil, similar to creating a panorama picture by splicing a series of smaller photographs together (Figure 5.21). Phased-array coils are not restricted to posterior positioning as for spine image, but are also used for scanning of anterior anatomy in abdominal or thoracic imaging. Several manufacturers have phased-array coils for examining other regions of the body (for example, head, neck, and knee).

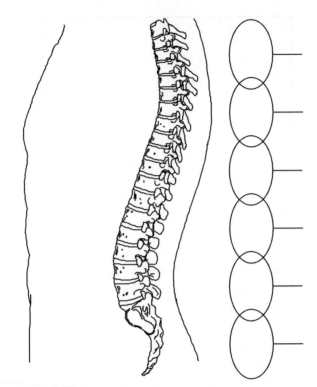

Figure 5.20 Phased-array coils. A large area such as the spine can be scanned using an array of smaller coils. The images from each coil can be combined to form the final image.

5.10 Parallel acquisition methods

In the description of phased-array coils above, each coil of the array is used to acquire a portion of the complete image, with the spatial resolution of each coil subimage equal to that of the final image. While the final image is produced by the combination of the subimages from the individual coils, each coil acquires minimal information away from its sensitive volume in the immediate area of the coil. Another application of phased-array coils uses the unique position of each coil within the array to augment the phase encoding process. This approach is used in so-called parallel acquisition methods. In the presence of G_{PE} in the appropriate direction, each coil experiences a different magnetic field $\boldsymbol{B}_i$ due to its location (equation (4.1)) and the spins that the coil senses will have different resonant frequencies (equation (4.2)). Rather than process the signal from each coil separately, the signals from all coils are merged to produce a single image prior to final processing. The measured signals are combined earlier in the image reconstruction process than with conventional phased-array coil imaging so that subimages from each coil are not representative of the final result; they are only

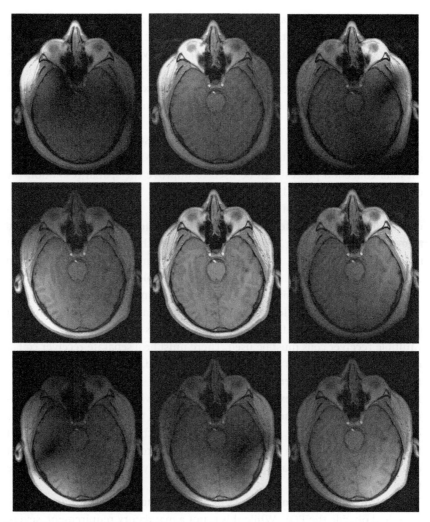

Figure 5.21 Images from the individual coils of an array (outer ring of images) can be combined to produce a single image (central image). Each outer image is sensitive to signals in its vicinity.

suitable when processed with the data from the other coils. This merger of signals enables fewer G_{PE} amplitudes to be used in the scan, so that the scan time can be reduced by a factor up to and including the number of coils used in the process, known as the acceleration factor.

This decrease in scan time is not without a penalty. The SNR is reduced for parallel acquisition techniques compared to the complete scan, with the SNR reduction greater for higher acceleration factors. This SNR reduction is attributed to two factors. The first is the simple fact that, by decreasing the sampling time, the SNR decreases as shown in equation (5.1). This reduced sampling time affects every voxel, so it leads to a uniform drop in SNR throughout the image. The second cause is known as the g-factor, or geometric factor. In voxels that are close to one coil but far from the other coils, it is relatively easy to "unmerge" the information, but it becomes difficult in voxels that are equidistant from all of the coils. This leads to a spatial variation in SNR where voxels near one of the receive coils will have a higher SNR than voxels that are approximately equidistant from all receive coils.

As a result, parallel acquisition techniques are most appropriate for scan protocols where the SNR is sufficiently high. In these circumstances, the more efficient data collection process can be used to improve the spatial resolution (by increasing N_{PE}), or reduce the scan time.

There are two classes of parallel techniques that are used in clinical scanning, based on when the merger of coil signals is performed: k-space-based and image-based (Figure 5.22). The difference between the techniques is the point during the data processing when the signals are combined. Both classes used increased ΔG_{PE} with fewer N_{PE} compared to a complete scan. Both classes are also computationally intensive, placing significant demands on the image reconstruction computer. Regardless of the method, there are four requirements that must be met to ensure that the data collection process does not induce artifacts:

1 Multiple receiver coils must be used. There must be a separate receiver coil at different spatial positions within the magnetic field. Most parallel acquisition techniques use phased-array coils.

2 Each receiver coil must experience a different B_i when G_{PE} is applied. This is easiest accomplished if the G_{PE} direction is parallel to the line connecting the coil centers (Figure 5.23). This is to ensure that each coil contributes different frequency components to the postprocessing. Failure to meet this requirement can potentially cause aliasing artifacts, which may be subtle or severe (see Chapter 9).

3 The FOV in both directions should be large enough so that minimal tissue is excited outside the FOV. While this is not a mandatory requirement, severe artifacts can occur if the FOV is significantly smaller than the anatomical region under observation.

4 The differences in individual coil sensitivities must be eliminated before the signal combination. If one coil is more sensitive than another due to hardware differences, then its contribution will be exaggerated in the final image, potentially causing artifacts. To eliminate this, calibration or reference scans are performed either prior to or during the primary scan that are used to compensate for the manufacturing imperfections.

The k-space-based parallel acquisition techniques merge the coil signals prior to Fourier transformation. In normal imaging, these higher harmonics produce aliasing artifacts (see Chapter 9). In the k-space-based techniques, the signals measured by the coils are not processed individually but are used to extract the correct (unaliased) signal from the combination signal (Figure 5.24).

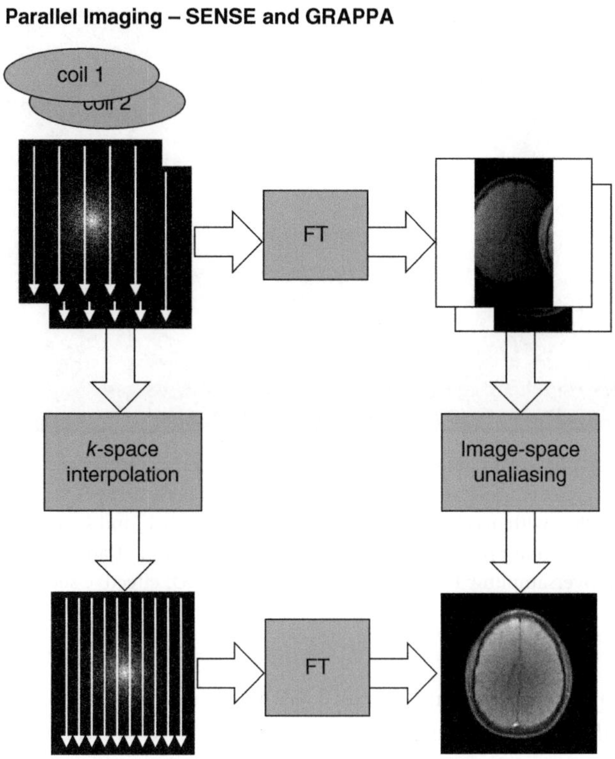

Parallel Imaging – SENSE and GRAPPA

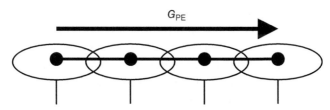

Figure 5.22 Principle of parallel imaging. A raw data set is acquired from each coil element. The data sets have a reduced number of lines, allowing for shorter measurement times. For k-space-based methods (solid lines), the raw data sets are combined to form a complete raw data set. The complete raw data set is processed to produce the final image. For image-based methods (dashed lines), the raw data sets are processed to produce images, and the images are combined to form the final image.

G_{PE}

Figure 5.23 The direction of G_{PE} should be aligned with the coil geometry axis. The different position of each coil means that the magnetic field will differ at each location.

Each element of the array will detect different amplitudes of the harmonics that are produced by a particular k_y line due to its different location. The coil geometry is such that sinusoidal patterns can be generated mathematically using linear combinations of the coil sensitivities, properly resolving the harmonics. Two k-space-based techniques are commonly used: SMASH (Simultaneous

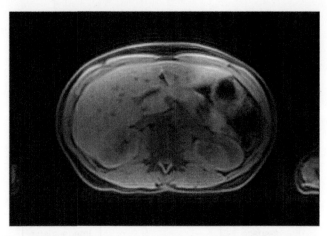

Figure 5.24 Three-dimensional transverse *T1*-weighted spoiled gradient echo image of abdomen with fat suppression, acquired using a 32-channel body array receiver coil. Scan parameters: GRAPPA with acceleration factors of 2 each in both k_y and k_z directions; *TR*, 4.9 ms; *TE*, 2.4 ms; excitation angle, 10°; acquisition matrix, N_{PE}, 131 and N_{RO}, 256 with twofold readout oversampling; FOV, 262 mm PE × 350 mm RO; effective slice thickness, 3.5 mm; time of acquisition, 8 s.

Acquisition of Spatial Harmonics) and GRAPPA (Generalized Autocalibrating Partially Parallel Acquisitions). The primary difference between them is when the calibration scans are acquired. SMASH acquires the calibration scans as a separate scan, enabling the primary scan time reduction to be directly proportional to the number of coils parallel to G_{PE}. The calibration scans can be used in multiple scans as long as the same coils are used. GRAPPA acquires the calibration scans as part of the primary scan. While this approach reduces the scan time savings, the calibration scans can be used in the final image as well, improving the SNR.

The other class of parallel acquisition techniques is image-based. The primary example of this approach is SENSE (Sensitivity Encoding). With SENSE, the number of k_y lines is reduced but Δk_y is increased so that the total span of *k*-space is maintained, effectively reducing FOV_{PH} for the image. An image is produced from the *k*-space sampled from each coil that contains both the correct image and the aliased portion due to the higher harmonics, but the amount of wrap at each spatial location is different for each coil. By comparing the different images and knowing the coil position and sensitivity, an unaliased image can be extracted from the different partial images.

CHAPTER 6

Pulse sequences

A pulse sequence is the measurement technique by which an MR image is obtained. It contains the hardware instructions (RF pulses, gradient pulses, and timings) necessary to acquire the data in the desired manner. As implemented by most manufacturers, the pulse sequence actually executed during the measurement is defined from parameters directly selected by the operator (e.g., *TR*, FOV) and variables defined in template files (e.g., basic relationships between RF pulses and slice selection gradients). This allows the operator to create a large number of pulse sequences using a limited number of template files. It also enables the manufacturer to limit parameter combinations to those suitable for execution. Some parameter limits of a pulse sequence (e.g., minimum *TR*, minimum FOV) depend on how the manufacturer has implemented the technique (e.g., gradient pulse duration), while other parameters (e.g., maximum gradient amplitude, gradient rise time) are determined by performance limits of the scanner hardware. The effect of common operator-selectable parameters on the signal intensity produced from a volume element of tissue is discussed in more detail in Chapter 7.

One of the more confusing aspects of MRI is the wide variety of pulse sequences available from the different equipment manufacturers and the even wider variety of pulse sequence names. In addition, similar sequences may be known by a variety of names by the same manufacturer. As a result, comparison of techniques and protocols between manufacturers is often difficult due to differences in sequence implementation. An accurate description and detailed comparison of techniques between manufacturers would require knowledge of proprietary information. Fortunately, there is an effort underway to provide a standardization of sequence nomenclature (DIN, 2008). This chapter describes several pulse sequences commonly used in imaging by all manufacturers and some of the general characteristics of each one. In addition, where appropriate, the common acronyms used by some of the major manufacturers for the sequences are included.

Comparison of pulse sequences is facilitated by the use of timing diagrams. Timing diagrams are schematic representations of the basic steps performed by the different hardware components during sequence execution. Although there

MRI Basic Principles and Applications, Fifth Edition.
Brian M. Dale, Mark A. Brown and Richard C. Semelka.
© 2015 John Wiley & Sons, Ltd. Published 2015 by John Wiley & Sons, Ltd.

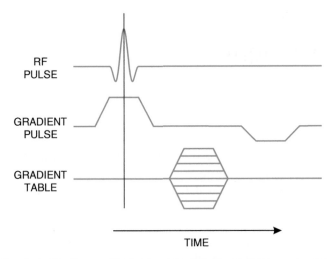

Figure 6.1 Simple timing diagram. The horizontal axis is time during sequence execution. Control signals for three hardware components are illustrated: the RF transmitter and two gradients (labeled RF Pulse, Gradient Pulse, and Gradient Table). The gradient pulse signals are executed the same way for each measurement, as indicated by the trapezoidal shape for the two gradient pulse waveforms. The gradient table signals change amplitude with each measurement and are represented by the multiple horizontal lines.

may be stylistic differences in the diagrams prepared by different authors, the general features are the same for all diagrams (Figure 6.1). Elapsed time during sequence execution is indicated from left to right along the horizontal axis. The vertical separation between lines is employed only for visualization. Each horizontal line corresponds to a different hardware component. At a minimum, four lines are used to describe any pulse sequence: one representing the radiofrequency (RF) transmitter and one representing each gradient (labeled as G_{SLICE}, G_{READ}, and G_{PHASE}, or G_X, G_Y, and G_Z). Additional lines may be added to indicate other activity such as analog-to-digital converter (ADC) sampling. Activity for a particular component such as a gradient pulse is shown as a deviation above or below the horizontal line (baseline). Simultaneous activity from more than one component such as the RF transmitter and slice selection gradient is indicated by nonzero activity from both lines at the same horizontal position. Constant-amplitude gradient pulses are shown as simple deviations from the baseline. Gradient tables such as for phase encoding are represented as hashed regions or sections with horizontal lines. Timing diagrams typically represent the hardware activity for the fundamental repeating unit of the pulse sequence, often called the kernel of the sequence. Specific details regarding exact timings, individual gradient amplitudes, or looping structures are not included as much of this information is determined by the specific measurement parameters or is proprietary to the various manufacturers. The generic nature of the representations makes timing diagrams suitable to represent classes of pulse sequences when making comparisons between the various measurement techniques.

6.1 Spin echo sequences

 A commonly used pulse sequence in MR imaging is a spin echo sequence. It has at least two RF pulses, an excitation pulse (often called the alpha (α) pulse) and one or more 180° refocusing pulses that generate the spin echo(es). A refocusing pulse is required for every echo produced. Spin echo sequences also utilize gradient pulses of opposite polarity in the readout and slice selection directions to refocus the protons at the same time as the spin echo; however, the contrast is determined primarily by the spin echo. Spoiler gradients are used following signal detection to dephase any residual transverse magnetization and minimize spurious echoes. In a spin echo sequence, the repetition time, TR, is the time between successive excitation pulses for a given slice. The echo time, TE, is the time from the excitation pulse to the echo maximum. A multislice loop structure is used to acquire signals from multiple slices within one TR time period. Table 6.1 lists some of the common names for spin echo sequences.

Table 6.1 Spin echo pulse sequence acronyms.

Siemens	GE	Philips
Single spin echo	Spin echo	Spin echo
Double echo	Multiecho multiplanar (MEMP)	Modified spin echo
Turbo spin echo (TSE)	Variable echo multiplanar (VEMP)	Multiple spin echo (MSE)
Half-Fourier acquisition turbo	Fast spin echo (FSE)	Turbo spin echo (TSE)
spin echo (HASTE)	Single-shot FSE (SS-FSE)	Ultra-fast spin echo (UFSE)

Three types of spin echo sequences are commonly used: standard single echo, standard multiecho, and echo train spin echo. Standard single echo sequences are generally used to produce $T1$-weighted images when acquired with relatively short TR and TE (less than 700 ms and 30 ms, respectively). A multislice loop structure is used with a single pair of excitation and refocusing pulses applied within the slice loop. A single phase encoding amplitude is applied per excitation pulse. Each echo within the scan is measured at the selected TE following application of a different amplitude for G_{PE} (Figure 6.2). A rectilinear, sequential filling of k-space is used. Following image reconstruction, amplitude variations between tissues in the image are the result of differences between tissue specific properties (proton density, $T1$, or $T2$).

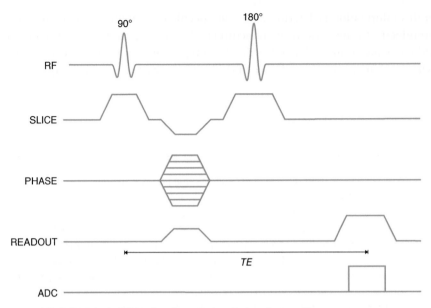

Figure 6.2 Standard single-echo spin echo sequence timing diagram. These sequences are characterized by a single 180° refocusing pulse, a single detected echo, and a single phase-encoding table. The *TE* time is measured from the middle of the excitation pulse to the center of the echo.

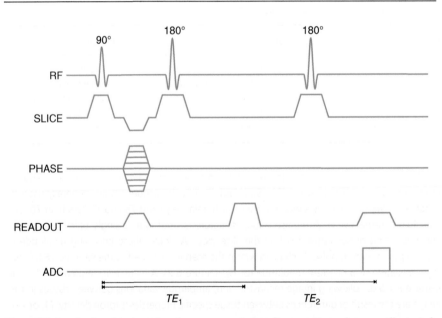

Figure 6.3 Standard multiecho spin echo sequence timing diagram. Two echoes are illustrated. Additional echoes may be generated by adding additional 180° RF pulses, slice-selection gradient pulses, readout gradient pulses, and ADC sampling period. Note the single phase-encoding gradient table. Both *TE* times are measured from the middle of the excitation pulse to the center of the respective echo.

Standard multiecho sequences apply multiple 180° refocusing RF pulses following a single excitation pulse. Each refocusing pulse produces a spin echo, each one at a different *TE* defined by the user. A single G_{PE} is used per RF excitation pulse (Figure 6.3). Differences in raw data signal intensity at each *TE* are still due to differences in G_{PE} only. This approach introduces raw data signal intensity variations from echo to echo (TE_1 to TE_2) due to *T2* relaxation. Images are created from the signals acquired at a single *TE* time. Multiecho sequences are used to produce proton density-weighted images using short *TE* (less than 30 ms) and *T2*-weighted images using long *TE* (greater than 80 ms) when *TR* is long enough to allow relatively complete *T1* relaxation for most tissues (2000 ms or longer).

The third type of spin echo sequence is known as the echo train spin echo (ETSE). It is based on the RARE (rapid acquisition with relaxation enhancement) technique for imaging. ETSE sequences are similar to standard multiecho sequences in that multiple 180° pulses are applied to produce multiple echoes following a single excitation pulse. However, each echo signal is acquired with a different G_{PE} as well as a different *TE* (Figure 6.4). The image is produced using some or all of the measured echoes as determined by the sequence design. The echo train length or turbo factor corresponds to the number of echoes used to create the image. A segmented filling of *k*-space is used with one echo from

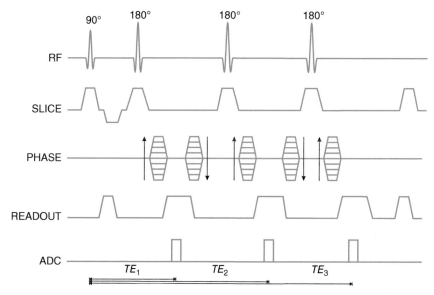

Figure 6.4 Echo train spin echo sequence timing diagram. A three-segment (echo train length of 3) version is illustrated, each with $N_{PE}/3$ values of G_{PE} per segment to acquire N_{PE} total lines of raw data. The arrows beside the G_{PE} tables indicate the direction in which the phase-encoding values change from one excitation pulse to the next. Gradient tables on opposite sides of the ADC sampling period have equal amplitudes but opposite polarity. The effective *TE* is the *TE* time (1, 2, or 3) during which the G_{PE} = 0 lines of data are acquired.

each segment acquired as part of the echo train for each RF pulse. The primary advantage of the ETSE technique is that the data collection process is more efficient and the scan time is reduced:

$$(\text{Scan time})_{ETSE} = TR * N_{SA} * N_{PE}/\text{Echo train length} \tag{6.1}$$

The contrast in ETSE sequences is determined primarily by the echoes detected at or near $G_{PE} = 0$ and the *TE*s for these echoes. The *TE* assigned to the image is referred to as an effective *TE* since there are echoes with different *TE*s contributing to the final image. This use of multiple *TE*s in the creation of the image makes ETSE sequences unsuitable for use when subtle differences in *T2* between tissues are responsible for the image contrast. Fat will also have an increased signal compared to standard spin echo or multiecho images acquired with the same *TE*.

While ETSE sequences can be used to produce *T1*-weighted images, their most common application has been to produce *T2*-weighted images. This is due to the significant reduction in scan time that can be achieved for long *TR* scans when modest echo train lengths are used. While echo train lengths less than 10 are typically used for brain and spine imaging, very long echo trains (100 or more) can be used in abdominal imaging to acquire *T2*-weighted images in less than one second. Termed snapshot or ultrafast ETSE, the scan times are sufficiently short to freeze bowel motion, yet provide good *T2* contrast between tissues.

6.2 Gradient echo sequences

Gradient echo sequences are a class of imaging techniques that do not use a 180° pulse to refocus the protons. The echo signal is generated only through gradient reversal. As mentioned in Chapter 3, application of imaging gradients induce proton dephasing. Application of a second gradient pulse of the same duration and magnitude but opposite polarity reverses this dephasing and produces an echo known as a gradient echo. All gradient echo sequences use gradient reversal pulses in at least two directions, the slice selection and the readout directions, which generate the echo signal. Excitation angles less than 90° are normally used (see Section 7.1).

The absence of the 180° RF pulse in gradient echo sequences has several important consequences. The sequence kernel time may be shorter than for an analogous spin echo sequence, enabling a shorter minimum *TR* or more slices to be acquired for the same *TR* if a multislice loop is used. Less total RF power is applied to the patient, so that the total RF energy deposition is lower. Additional contrast mechanisms are also possible. The static sources for proton dephasing, B_0 inhomogeneity, and magnetic susceptibility differences contribute to the signal decay, so the *TE* determines the amount of *T2** weighting in a gradient echo image rather than only *T2* weighting as in a spin echo image (equation (3.2)). For this reason, the overall signal level in gradient echo images will be less than for spin echo images with comparable acquisition parameters. The image quality of gradient echo sequences is also more sensitive to metal implants and to the region of anatomy under investigation. In addition, fat and water protons within a voxel also contribute different amounts of signal, depending upon the chosen *TE*, a process known as phase cycling (see Chapter 9, Phase cancellation artifact). Table 6.2 lists some of the common gradient echo sequences currently in use.

Table 6.2   Gradient echo pulse sequence acronyms.

Siemens	GE	Philips
Fast low angle shot (FLASH)	Spoiled GRASS (SPGR), fast spoiled GRASS (FSPGR), multiplanar spoiled GRASS (MPSPGR), fast multiplanar spoiled GRASS (FMPSPGR)	*T1* contrast-enhanced FFE (*T1* CE-FFE)
Fast imaging with steady-state precession (FISP), true FISP	Gradient acquisition in the steady state (GRASS), fast GRASS, multiplanar GRASS (MPGR), fast multiplanar GRASS (FMPGR), FIESTA	Fast field echo (FFE)
Reversed FISP (PSIF)	Steady-state free precession (SSFP)	*T2* contrast-enhanced FFE (*T2* CE-FFE)
TurboFLASH, magnetization prepared rapid acquisition gradient echo (MP-RAGE)	IR-prepared fast GRASS, driven equilibrium (DE)-prepared fast GRASS	Turbo field echo (TFE)

The simplest gradient echo sequence is a spoiled gradient echo sequence. This sequence uses a spoiling scheme to dephase the transverse magnetization following signal detection. As a result, only longitudinal magnetization contributes to *M* at the time of the next excitation pulse. Spoiling may be done either by applying high amplitude gradient pulses known as "spoiler" or "crusher" gradients to dephase the magnetization or by varying the phase of the RF excitation pulse in a pseudorandom fashion following each application. This approach, known as RF spoiling, produces an incoherent addition of any residual transverse magnetization so that the only remaining coherence at the time of the next excitation pulse is in the longitudinal direction (Figure 6.5).

In many respects, spoiled gradient echo sequences are the gradient echo counterpart of spin echo sequences. However, the contrast behavior of spoiled gradient echo techniques is slightly more complicated. The *TE* determines the amount of *T2** rather than *T2* weighting. The combination of excitation angle and *TR* determines the amount of *T1* weighting. Low excitation angle pulses impart minimal RF energy and leave most of *M* in the longitudinal direction. This allows a shorter *TR* to be used without producing saturation of the protons. Proton density-weighted images are produced for small excitation angles (15–20°), relatively long *TR* (500 ms), and short *TE* (<10 ms). *T2** weighted images can be obtained using the same excitation angle and *TR* but a long *TE*

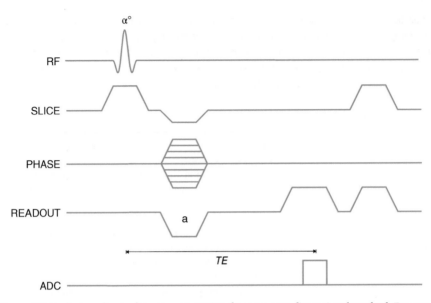

Figure 6.5 Spoiled gradient echo sequence timing diagram, two-dimensional method. Because there is no 180° RF pulse, the polarity of the G_{RO} dephasing gradient pulse (a) is opposite that of the readout gradient pulse applied during signal detection. Gradient spoiling is illustrated at the end of the kernel. The *TE* time is measured from the middle of the excitation pulse to the center of the echo.

(25–30 ms). Substantial *T1* weighting is obtained using large excitation angles (80° or greater), short *TR* (100–150 ms), and short *TE* (<10 ms).

Spoiled gradient echo images may be acquired using any of the sequence looping techniques discussed in Chapter 4. Routine spoiled gradient echo imaging for spinal or abdominal studies uses a 2D multislice mode. A 2D sequential mode is used for MR angiography (see Chapter 11) while a 3D volume acquisition can produce very thin slices useful for multiplanar reconstruction of images in arbitrary orientations.

A second group of gradient sequences belongs to a class of techniques known as refocused or steady-state gradient echo sequences. Refocused gradient echo sequences use a single excitation pulse with a *TR* shorter than the *T2* relaxation time and do not use spoiling. Once *M* has reached a steady-state value (following a few RF pulses), both longitudinal and transverse components are present at the time of the next excitation pulse. Unlike spoiled gradient echo sequences, refocused sequences apply rephasing gradient pulses in one, two, or all three directions to maintain the transverse magnetization as much as possible. In addition, the excitation pulses are applied rapidly enough (short *TR*) so that spin echoes are generated that occur simultaneously with the subsequent excitation pulses. These spin echoes refocus the transverse magnetization as in spin echo imaging so that the signal amplitude in refocused pulse sequences depends strongly upon the *T1* and *T2* relaxation times of the tissues under observation. Optimal contrast can only be achieved in tissues with long *T1* and *T2* relaxation times.

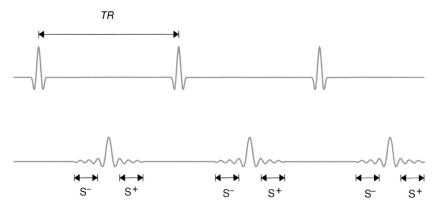

Figure 6.6 A series of equally spaced RF pulses produces spin echoes that form at the time of the subsequent RF excitation pulses. Once a steady state is reached (following several *TR* time periods), signal is induced prior to and following the excitation pulse. The preexcitation pulse signal (S⁻) is strictly echo reformation. The postexcitation pulse signal (S⁺) is a combination of echo and free induction decay. Images can be produced from either signal or from both.

Two signals can be measured from a refocused pulse scheme, one before and one after the refocusing pulse (Figure 6.6). This scenario is analogous to examining a normal spin echo and using the protons as they rephase prior to *TE* to produce one signal and as they dephase following *TE* to produce the other signal. In spin echo imaging, both halves of the echo are detected and are processed together. In gradient echo imaging, each half of the echo can produce an image. The two pulse sequences are complementary in their sequence timing (Figure 6.7). The technique using the postexcitation pulse signal is conceptually similar to the spoiled gradient echo technique except for the unspoiled transverse magnetization.

Bright signals are produced by both pre- and postexcitation techniques for tissues such as cerebrospinal fluid and blood with relatively long *T2* values and when *TR* is short so that the transverse coherence is maintained. A difference between the two techniques is observed when using a long *TR* or for tissues with *T2* that is much shorter than *T1*. In general, the postexcitation S⁺ signal in Figure 6.6 is based on net magnetization derived from two sources present at the time of the RF excitation pulse: the transverse magnetization M_T produced by previous excitation pulses, which generates a spin echo and decays based on *T2* relaxation, and the longitudinal magnetization M_L resulting from *T1* relaxation, which generates an FID and decays based on *T2**.

Elimination of this M_T component is accomplished in two ways. The use of spoiling, either gradient-based or RF-based, explicitly removes this component as in spin echo sequences. Use of a long *TR* (e.g., 500 ms) with a small excitation pulse angle (10–15°) allows this component to decay naturally. In both approaches, only the M_L component is present, so that the decay of S⁺ is based on *T2**. This means that equivalent contrast results are obtained for spoiled and refocused gradient echo techniques if a long *TR* and low excitation pulse angle

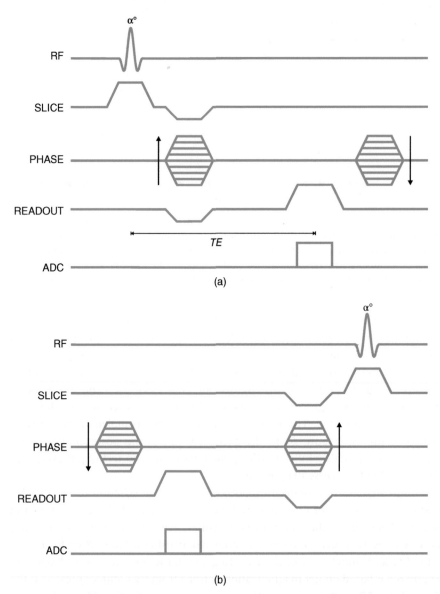

Figure 6.7 Refocused gradient echo sequence timing diagrams. Instead of spoiling the transverse magnetization, rephasing gradients are used to maintain the transverse magnetization as much as possible. (a) Postexcitation imaging sequence; (b) preexcitation imaging sequence.

are used. For the preexcitation technique, the signal is derived from the M_T component only so that, with spoiling or using long *TR*, no image is produced.

For refocused gradient echo sequences using short *TR* and a large excitation pulse angle, the presence of the M_T component in S^+ increases the signal from tissue with long *T2* such as fluid. The problem is that the two resulting transverse

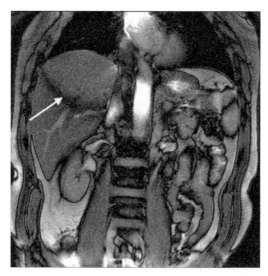

Figure 6.8 Coronal image acquired with fully refocused gradient echo technique. The arrow indicates a signal cancellation artifact due to interference between the pre-and postexcitation signals. (Reproduced with permission of H. Cecil Charles, Duke University.)

magnetizations can decay at different rates, particularly if the magnet homogeneity is not uniform. This causes a phase difference in those tissues to develop and can result in an interference banding artifact appearing in the postexcitation images if there is a significant signal from the M_T component (Figure 6.8). The use of refocusing gradients retains this component as much as possible, but the extent of banding increases with increased refocusing. Use of complete gradient refocusing (so-called steady-state free precession sequences) should be preceded by adjustment of the magnet homogeneity. This will increase the $T2*$ for the M_L-based signal and will reduce the extent of banding.

6.3 Echo planar imaging sequences

A third type of pulse sequence, echo planar imaging (EPI), uses a very different method for data collection. EPI sequences are characterized by a series of gradient reversals in the readout direction. Each reversal produces a gradient echo, with the second half of one readout period being rephased by the first half of the subsequent readout period. The gradient reversals are performed very rapidly, allowing echo planar images to be acquired in 100–200 ms. Two types of schemes are used to phase encode each gradient echo. The continuous phase encoding method typically used on older hardware applies the phase encoding gradient continuously throughout the readout period. If a preparatory phase encoding pulse is applied, then each echo is acquired with a different amount of total phase accumulation; that is, k-space is sampled in a continuous and sinusoidal fashion (Figure 6.9a).

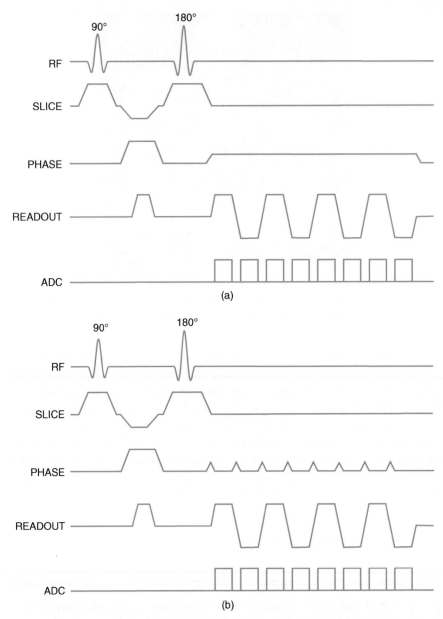

Figure 6.9 Echo planar imaging sequence timing diagrams. A spin echo excitation scheme and an echo train length of 8 are illustrated. (a) Constant phase encoding. The phase-encoding gradient is on for the entire data collection period. Each data point of each echo has a unique amount of G_{PE} influence. (b) Blipped phase encoding. The phase-encoding gradient is applied incrementally prior to detection of each echo. Each echo is influenced by a different amount of G_{PE}, but each data point within the echo has the same amount of G_{PE} influence.

Regridding in one or both directions (Section 5.4) is necessary to ensure a k-space of uniform density. Alternately, a "blipped" phase encoding technique used on most modern systems applies a small amplitude G_{PE} pulse (equal to Δk_y) prior to each sampling period. No phase encoding gradient is applied during signal detection so that the phase encoding for each echo is constant (Figure 6.9b). The raw data matrix is acquired in a rectilinear, zigzag fashion. Because of the use of gradient echoes, EPI sequences are very sensitive to $T2^*$ effects. In particular, magnetic susceptibility differences will cause image distortions at tissue–bone or tissue–air interfaces, making their use problematic in some anatomical regions.

Two data collection schemes are used in EPI sequences: single-shot and segmented or multishot. Single-shot techniques acquire all phase encoding steps following a single excitation pulse. Since only one RF pulse is applied per slice position, each image can be acquired with an "infinite" TR. Modern gradient amplifiers may be required for single-shot EPI imaging because of the rapid switching of the readout gradient polarity necessary to acquire all the echoes. Segmented techniques acquire a subset of phase-encoding steps following each excitation pulse. A segmented loop structure with multiple excitation pulses is used to acquire all phase encoding steps. Segmented EPI can often be performed with older imaging gradient systems.

The contrast in EPI images is determined by the TE for the echo acquired when $k_y = 0$. Each echo is acquired at a different TE similar to echo train spin echo sequences, so the TE of the image is referred to as an effective TE. Variations in contrast for EPI sequences are achieved using magnetization-preparation pulses (see Section 6.4) applied prior to the readout period. $T1$-weighted images are produced using a 180° inversion RF pulse prior to the excitation pulse. $T2$-weighted images can be obtained using a 90–180° pair of pulses to produce a spin echo. Spoiled gradient echo EPI sequences use no preparatory pulse and produce $T2^*$-weighted images.

6.4 Magnetization-prepared sequences

The pulse sequences described previously provide the fundamental methods used for spatial localization in MRI today. For certain combinations of measurement parameters, the images that result from these techniques may have a lack of tissue contrast or poor spatial resolution. In order to overcome these limitations, the basic techniques may be modified using RF pulses to preset the net magnetization to a given state prior to execution of the spatial localization steps. These extra pulses are known as magnetization-preparation pulses and the sequences that incorporate them are collectively known as magnetization-prepared (MP) sequences.

One example of an MP sequence is known as inversion recovery (IR). The traditional IR sequence is a variation of the spin echo sequence. It is a spin echo sequence with an additional 180° pulse, usually slice-selective, applied prior to the initial excitation pulse. The 180° pulse inverts **M** for the protons within the slice, producing enhanced *T1* sensitivity at the time of the excitation pulse. The inversion time, *TI*, is a user-selectable delay time between the 180° pulse and the excitation pulse and determines the amount of *T1* relaxation that occurs between the two pulses. A standard phase encoding gradient table is used, and *TE* is defined as for spin echo sequences (Figure 6.10). Table 6.3 lists common names and features for inversion recovery sequences. Inversion recovery sequences require long *TR* times to allow maximal *T1* relaxation between successive excitation RF pulses. Insufficient *TR* causes loss of signal due to saturation for tissues with long *T1* relaxation times such as fluids.

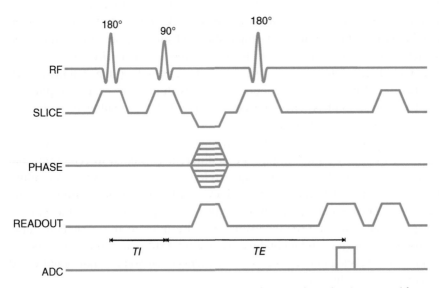

Figure 6.10 Standard inversion recovery sequence timing diagram. The *TI* time is measured from the center of the inversion (initial 180°) pulse to the center of the excitation pulse. The *TE* time is measured from the center of the excitation pulse to the center of the echo.

Table 6.3 Inversion recovery pulse sequence acronyms.

Siemens	GE	Philips
Standard inversion recovery	Multiplanar IR (MPIR)	IR
Echo train inversion recovery	Fast multiplanar IR (FMPIR)	IR-turbo spin echo (IR-TSE)
Interleaved excitation	Nonsequential (standard)	
Magnitude reconstruction	Absolute value, magnitude	Modulus real
Phase-sensitive reconstruction		

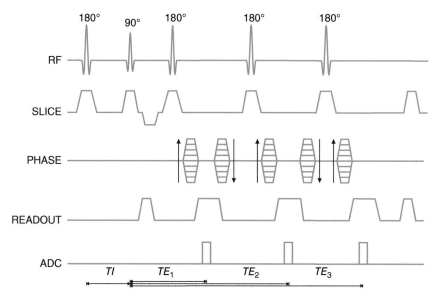

Figure 6.11 Echo train inversion recovery sequence timing diagram. A three-segment (echo train length of 3) version is illustrated, each segment with $N_{PE}/3$ values for G_{PE}. The TI time is measured from the center of the inversion (initial 180°) pulse to the excitation pulse. The effective TE is the TE time (1, 2, or 3) during which the $G_{PE} = 0$ lines of data are acquired.

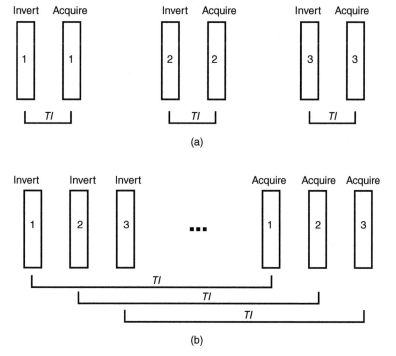

Figure 6.12 Inversion recovery looping modes. (a) Inversion for a given slice is followed immediately by echo acquisition. This is typically used when the TI time is relatively short. (b) All inversion pulses for all slices are performed followed by echo acquisition. This is typically used when the TI time is relatively long.

IR pulses can be used in conjunction with all the sequence types mentioned previously. Their most frequent usage is with ETSE sequences, although their use with gradient echo or EPI sequences is also relatively common. The echo train inversion recovery sequence combines features of the normal IR and the ETSE sequences. The 180° inversion pulse is applied prior to an ETSE acquisition sequence rather than a normal spin echo sequence. The contrast obtained in an echo train IR sequence is based on the *TI* and the tissue *T1* times as in the IR sequence, while the echo train length and effective *TE* have equivalent effects to these parameters in the ETSE sequence (Figure 6.11). The second modification is the looping mode for multislice imaging. If the *TI* time is relatively short, all RF pulses are applied and the signal is detected from a slice before progressing to another slice. If the *TI* time is relatively long, all inversion RF pulses are applied in order, followed by the excitation and refocusing pulses and signal detection. This provides for more efficient data collection during one *TR* time period (Figure 6.12).

The image reconstruction process will have a significant role in the appearance of IR-type images. The inversion of M by the 180° RF pulse allows for the generation of negative amplitude signals. Short *TI* times allow minimal *T1* relaxation between the inversion and excitation RF pulses. Most tissues will have M inverted at the time of the excitation pulse. Long *TI* times allow more complete relaxation of tissues between the two pulses to occur, producing positive values for M. Intermediate *TI* gives a mixture of positive and negative M, depending on *TI* and the specific tissue *T1* values (Figure 6.13). During image reconstruction, the phase of M can be incorporated into the pixel intensity. Termed phase-sensitive IR, these images have negative pixel values for tissues with inverted M. These are produced by tissues with long *TI* values at short *TI* times. Background air is assigned a midrange pixel value. Phase-sensitive IR images have the largest range of pixel values of any imaging technique. Alternately, the phase of M can be ignored in the final image. Termed absolute value or magnitude IR, these images have pixel values based only on the signal magnitude. Tissues with very short or very long *T1* relaxation times have high pixel values and background air has a low pixel value (Figure 6.14).

The inversion pulse also enables the suppression of signal through the proper choice of *TI*. If the *TI* time is chosen so that the tissue of interest has no longitudinal component at the time of the excitation pulse, then that tissue contributes no signal to the final image. This time, known as the null time for the tissue, is determined by the *T1* relaxation time for the tissue:

$$TI_{NULL} = 0.693 * T1 \qquad (6.2)$$

assuming that the *TR* time is sufficiently long. The two most common applications of IR sequences are for the suppression of cerebrospinal fluid (CSF) and fat. Normal CSF has a *T1* relaxation time of approximately 3000 ms at 1.5 T. A *TI* time of 2080 ms applies the excitation pulse when the CSF magnetization has no longitudinal component and produces an image with no CSF signal. This technique,

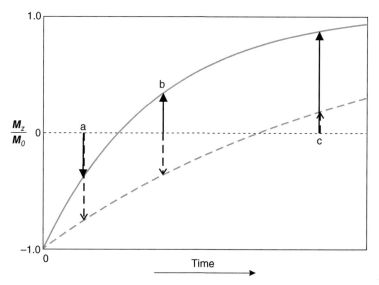

Figure 6.13 *TI* recovery curves for inversion recovery sequences. The 180° inversion pulse inverts the net magnetization for all tissues. Tissue with a short *TI* time (solid curve) recovers faster than tissue with a long *TI* (dashed curve) time. For a *TI* time of (a), both tissues contribute significant negative amplitude signal. For a *TI* time of (b), the short *TI* tissue contributes positive amplitude signal while the long *TI* tissue contributes negative amplitude signal. For a *TI* time of (c), the short *TI* tissue contributes significant positive amplitude signal and the long *TI* tissue contributes minimal signal. If the signal polarity is considered (phase-sensitive IR sequences), signal difference will be seen at all three *TI* times. If the signal polarity is ignored (absolute value or magnitude IR sequences), no difference in signal between the two tissues will be seen at time (b).

known as fluid-attenuated IR (FLAIR), allows easy visualization of gray and white matter inflammation.

Fat has a heterogeneous structure and its signal is a composite of all the tissue types within it. It has a *TI* relaxation time of approximately 200–250 ms at 1.5 T. If a *TI* value of 140–160 ms is selected, the excitation pulse occurs when the fat magnetization has no longitudinal component and produces an image with no fat signal. This technique is known as STIR, or short *TI* inversion recovery. Virtually complete and uniform fat suppression throughout the imaging volume can be achieved using STIR imaging using the correct *TI*. However, it suffers from two major limitations. One is that the sequence kernel time is longer due to the *TI* time. As a result, a limited number of slices can be acquired for a typical *TR*. Complete coverage of the desired anatomical region may require the use of multiple scans or the ETSE sequence variation. The second problem occurs when using a *TI* contrast agent. As described in Chapter 15, gadolinium-based contrast agents such as Gd-DTPA shorten the *TI* relaxation time for the water in tissues that absorb the agent. Tissues with long *TI* values that would normally be bright in a STIR image will lose signal if the contrast agent is present as the tissue

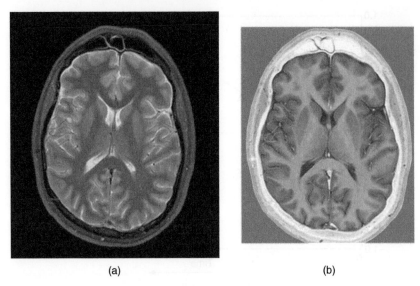

(a)   (b)

Figure 6.14 Magnitude (a) and phase-sensitive (b) inversion recovery images. All other measurement parameters are equal: pulse sequence, echo train spin echo, five echoes; *TR*, 7000 ms; *TE*, 14 ms; *TI*, 140 ms; acquisition matrix; N_{PE}, 224 and N_{RO}, 256; *FOV*, 201 mm PE × 230 mm RO; N_{SA}, 1; slice thickness, 5 mm.

T1 approaches that of the fat tissue. Visualization of these tissues thus becomes difficult. For this reason, STIR imaging is usually not performed when contrast agents are administered.

MP pulses can also be incorporated into gradient echo and EPI sequences. These pulses are often used to improve tissue contrast for scans where short measurement times are desired. For example, a *TR* of 7 ms with $N_{PE} = 128$ will require 900 ms of scan time. The excitation angle must be between 5° and 10° to minimize saturation effects yet produce sufficient transverse magnetization to generate a signal. Added contrast may be obtained by manipulating the longitudinal magnetization through the application of additional RF pulses prior to the gradient echo sequence. These preparation pulses generate enhanced amplitude variations to *M* that can be measured during the rapid data collection time. This is the concept of MP gradient echo sequences. The same approach is used for single-shot EPI sequences. An inversion pulse is added prior to the excitation to provide *T1* weight. The *TI* time is the primary parameter that controls the amount of *T1* influence.

One major difference between the usage of MP pulses in gradient echo or EPI sequences compared to spin echo-based sequences is in the frequency of application of the MP pulse. Spin echo-based sequences apply one MP pulse per excitation pulse so that the MP-modified net magnetization has a steady-state value for the scan. In other words, the modified *M* will be constant at the time of the excitation pulse, though different from its value in the absence of the MP pulse. EPI sequences also apply one MP pulse per excitation pulse, but they are non-steady-state techniques since M does not have the same value prior to each phase encoding step due to the EPI data collection process.

Gradient echo sequences typically apply a single MP pulse followed by multiple excitation pulses. As a result, gradient echo MP techniques are also non-steady-state techniques since M does not have the same value prior to each phase encoding step. Each phase encoding step is acquired at a different point in time following the preparation pulses. The resulting image contrast depends on when the $G_{PE} = 0$ step is acquired during the data collection period. The $G_{PE} = 0$ time is determined by the particular gradient table-ordering scheme used. Linear k-space ordering has the $k_y = 0$ line in the middle of the phase encoding table so that the contrast-controlling echoes are acquired at a time $TR * N_{PE} *N_{SA}/2$ into the data collection period (see Figure 5.10). The contrast in this case depends on the matrix size and acquisitions. Centric ordering acquires the $G_{PE} = 0$ step at the beginning of the data collection period so that the $G_{PE} = 0$ step occurs at a time TR into the data collection period (see Figure 5.14). The contrast for a centric-ordered magnetization prepared sequence does not vary as dramatically with the extrinsic variables and has a more predictable contrast behavior.

Two types of RF preparatory schemes are used in MP gradient echo sequences. As mentioned previously, $T1$-weighted images can be produced applying a single 180° inversion RF pulse prior to the data collection (Figure 6.15). This pulse may be nonselective to invert all protons within the transmitter coil or slice selective

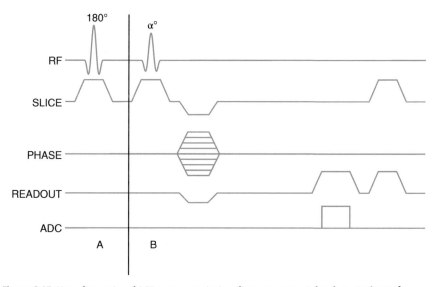

Figure 6.15 Two-dimensional MP sequence timing diagram, $T1$-weighted. A single 180° inversion RF pulse is applied once per scan (section A). This inversion provides significant $T1$ weighting to M. The portion of the sequence indicated by B is repeated for the N_{SA} and N_{PE} desired.

to invert only the protons in the slice of interest. A delay time *TI* between the inversion pulse and the data collection period produces variation in longitudinal magnetization of the tissues. *T1* MP sequences differ from the IR sequences described previously in that only one inversion pulse is applied for the entire data collection period. The contrast is determined by the effective *TI*, which is the time between the inversion and the $k_y = 0$ line:

$$TI_{effective} = TI + TR * N_{SA} * N_{PE}/2 \tag{6.3}$$

For *T2* MP gradient echo sequences, a series of RF pulses known as a driven equilibrium pulse train is used. Three equally spaced RF pulses are applied with amplitudes 90°–τ–180°–τ–90° (Section A in Figure 6.16). The first two pulses generate a spin echo and produce *T2* weighting to the transverse magnetization. The third pulse rotates this magnetization into the longitudinal direction, producing changes in **M** based on the *T2* relaxation times and the interpulse spacing τ. Use of a centric-ordered data collection produces *T2*-weighted images with good contrast.

MP gradient echo sequences can be either 2D or 3D techniques. Two-dimensional magnetization prepared techniques are acquired as sequential slice techniques in that all data collection is acquired for a slice following a single set of preparation pulses. The rapid measurement times make them very

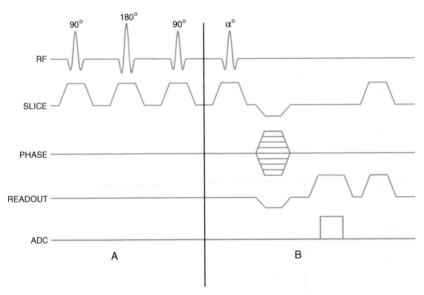

Figure 6.16 Two-dimensional MP sequence timing diagram, T2-weighted. A 90°– 180°– 90° RF pulse train is applied once prior to the data collection scheme (section A). The first two pulses produce T2 weighting to **M**, which is restored to the longitudinal direction by the final pulse prior to the data collection. The portion of the sequence indicated by B is repeated for the N_{SA} and N_{PE} desired.

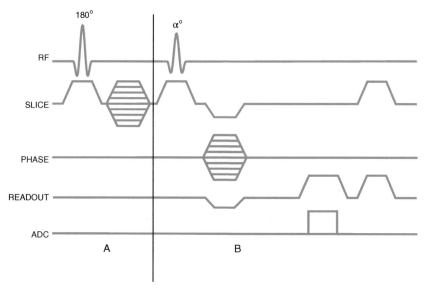

Figure 6.17 Three-dimensional MP sequence timing diagram, *T1*-weighted. A 180° inversion RF pulse is applied followed by encoding in the slice (k_z) direction (section A). This inversion provides significant *T1* weighting to **M**. The portion of the sequence indicated by *B* is repeated for the N_{PE} desired. The entire process (A and B) is repeated for the N_{SA} and N_{PAR} desired.

insensitive to patient motion. These sequences may also be acquired using a segmented *k*-space in order to increase spatial resolution. Three-dimensional MP techniques typically apply one MP pulse per phase encoding entry (k_y) so that the non-steady-state behavior to **M** is only present during the loop through the partitions gradient table (k_z) (Figure 6.17). This approach enables the image contrast to be unaffected by the acquisition matrix. It also reduces the number of measured values of *M* as the number of k_z values is normally smaller than the number of k_y values.

CHAPTER 7

Measurement parameters and image contrast

As mentioned in Chapter 6, many of the measurement parameters of a pulse sequence may be modified through the user interface software. The particular parameters will be determined by the scanner manufacturer, based on the template pulse sequence (which parameters are appropriate for modification) and the desired interface design (which parameters should the operator be allowed to modify). There are three general criteria that should be considered when modifying any measurement parameter as described in Chapter 5: acceptable scan time, adequate spatial resolution, and sufficient contrast between tissues relative to the background noise (contrast-to-noise ratio). These criteria are often in conflict in clinical imaging. For example, obtaining images with high spatial resolution (pixel sizes < 0.7 mm) and high contrast-to-noise ratio between tissues will require long scan times due to signal averaging. For each scan, the important criterion must be identified so that appropriate parameter variations can be made. One complication is that, while the scan time and spatial resolution for the final image can be calculated before the scan begins, the contrast-to-noise ratio cannot be determined prior to the measurement. This is because the measured signal amplitude depends on the specific tissue(s) within the imaging volume and their relaxation times. Another complication is that the most important criterion may change, depending on the anatomical region under observation. For example, imaging of the central nervous system will normally have scans with longer measurement times so that higher spatial resolution and contrast-to-noise ratios can be obtained. By comparison, to reduce motion, imaging of the thoracic or abdominal cavity employs scans with short measurement times and will compromise on the spatial resolution and contrast-to-noise ratio to achieve them.

As mentioned above, the specific parameters that are variable within the user interface and their specific definitions will be determined by the manufacturer. However, many parameters are commonly available in most pulse sequences. One approach to categorizing them is by their effect on the final image. Intrinsic parameters modify the inherent signal produced by a volume element of tissue (voxel). These parameters probe the characteristic tissue properties that are

---

MRI Basic Principles and Applications, Fifth Edition.
Brian M. Dale, Mark A. Brown and Richard C. Semelka.

the response to the measurement procedure. Intrinsic parameters affect only the signal-producing portion of the image, which is normally patient anatomy and not background air. Extrinsic parameters influence the mechanics of data collection (e.g., voxel size) or other factors external to the tissue. They typically affect the spatial resolution or general background noise levels in the final image. Many of these parameters are specific to the particular choice of pulse sequence used for the measurement and may not be available in all instances. The definitions below are the common ones for these parameters.

7.1 Intrinsic parameters

Repetition time, *TR*, measured in ms, is the time between successive RF excitation pulses applied to a given volume of tissue. In conjunction with the excitation angle (see following), *TR* determines the amount of *T1* weighting contributing to the image contrast. If all other factors are equal, longer *TR* allows more time for the RF excitation energy to be dissipated by the protons through spin-lattice relaxation, producing images with less *T1* weighting (Figure 7.1). For a multislice loop, *TR* limits the number of slices that can be acquired during the measurement.

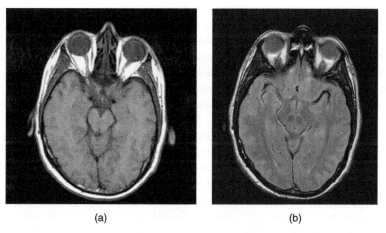

(a)   (b)

Figure 7.1 *TR* effects on image contrast. Longer *TR* allows more time for *T1* relaxation and produces more signal from tissues with long *T1* values. Other measurement parameters are: pulse sequence, spin echo; *TE*, 30 ms; acquisition matrix, N_{PE}, 224 and N_{RO}, 256; FOV, 201 mm PE × 230 mm RO; N_{SA}, 1; slice thickness, 5 mm. (a) *TR* of 500 ms; (b) *TR* of 2000 ms. Note reversal of contrast between gray matter and white matter in (b) compared to (a).

Echo time, *TE*, measured in ms, is the time between the excitation pulse and the echo (signal maximum). It determines the amount of *T2* weighting for spin echo images (Figure 7.2). For gradient echo images, *TE* determines the amount of *T2** weighting and the ratio of fat and

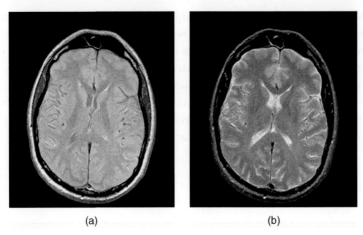

(a)   (b)

Figure 7.2 *TE* effects on image contrast. Longer *TE* allows more time for *T2* relaxation and produces more signal from tissues with long *T2* values. Other measurement parameters are: pulse sequence, spin echo; *TR*, 2000 ms; acquisition matrix, N_{PE}, 224 and N_{RO}, 256; FOV, 201 mm PE × 230 mm RO; N_{SA}, 1; slice thickness, 5 mm. (a) *TE* of 30 ms; (b) *TE* of 80 ms. Note bright signal from cerebrospinal fluid (CSF) in (b) compared to (a).

water signal contributions (see Figure 2.6). Longer *TE* allows more time for proton dephasing and produces lower signal amplitudes. In echo train spin echo, echo planar imaging, and MP gradient echo sequences, *TE* is considered to be effective since all echoes used in image reconstruction are not acquired at the same echo time.

Inversion time, *TI*, measured in ms, is the time between the 180° inversion pulse and the imaging excitation pulse. *TI* is used in inversion recovery (IR), echo train IR, and magnetization-prepared gradient echo sequences, and determines the amount of time allowed for *T1* relaxation following the inversion pulse. Short TI times allow minimum *T1* relaxation, while long *TI* times allow significant *T1* relaxation prior to the imaging excitation pulse. Proper choice of *TI* enables signal suppression of tissues based on their *T1* relaxation times (Figure 7.3).

Echo train length (also known as the turbo factor) is the number of echoes (number of phase encoding steps) measured following an excitation pulse that are used to create an image. The echo train length is used in echo train spin echo, echo train IR, and echo planar sequences. For long *TR*, longer echo train lengths allow shorter scan times through more efficient data collection. The sequence kernel time (minimum *TR* per slice) is longer with longer echo train lengths, producing greater signal attenuation in the late echoes through *T2* relaxation as well as requiring a longer minimum *TR* to obtain an equal number of slices. The number of phase encoding steps for the measurement is a multiple of the echo train length.

Echo spacing, measured in ms, is the time between each echo of the echo train. The echo spacing is used in ETSE, echo train IR, and echo planar sequences. Longer echo spacing allows more time for *T2* relaxation between each echo. Shorter echo spacing reduces the sequence kernel time.

The excitation angle (also known as the flip angle), measured in degrees, is the amount of rotation away from the equilibrium axis that ***M*** undergoes through RF absorption. If not variable under the operating software, the excitation angle is usually 90° in order to generate the maximum transverse magnetization. The excitation angle is also proportional to the amount

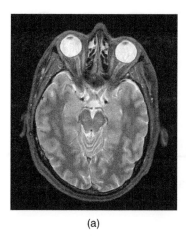
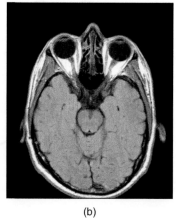

(a)   (b)

Figure 7.3 *TI* effects on image contrast. Longer *TI* allows more time for *T1* relaxation following the inversion pulse. The choice of *TI* can cause signal suppression of different tissues. Other measurement parameters are: pulse sequence, echo train spin echo, five echoes; *TR*, 7000 ms; *TE*, 14 ms; acquisition matrix, N_{PE}, 224 and N_{RO}, 256; FOV, 201 mm PE × 230 mm RO; N_{SA}, 1; slice thickness, 5 mm. (a) *TI* = 140 ms (fat suppression); (b) *TI* = 2100 ms (CSF suppression).

of energy absorbed and the amount of signal produced by the protons. The excitation angle, together with *TR* and the *T1* values for the individual tissues, determines the amount of *T1* weighting present in an image. For gradient echo sequences, the Ernst angle α_E is the excitation angle that produces the maximum signal from a tissue for a particular *TR*:

$$\cos(\alpha_E) = \exp(-TR/T1) \tag{7.1}$$

7.2 Extrinsic parameters

Slice thickness, *TH*, measured in mm, is the volume of tissue in the slice selection direction that absorbs the RF energy during excitation and generates the signal. Variation in slice thickness is usually accomplished through changing the magnitude of G_{SS}. Thicker slices provide more signal per voxel whereas thinner slices produce less partial volume averaging.

Slice gap, measured in mm, is the space between adjacent slices. The slice gap may also be expressed as a fraction of the slice thickness, depending on the operating software. The slice gap allows the user to control the size of the total imaging volume by increasing or decreasing the space between slices. The slice gap also provides a method to compensate for the imperfect RF excitation pulses. If the slices are closely spaced, excitation pulses applied to adjacent slice position partially overlap and excite the same region of tissue because the slice excitation profiles are not uniform. This situation is known as crosstalk (Figure 7.4). Due to the rapid RF pulse application, these regions of overlap become saturated

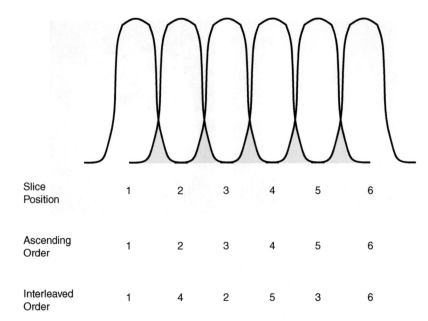

Slice Position	1	2	3	4	5	6
Ascending Order	1	2	3	4	5	6
Interleaved Order	1	4	2	5	3	6

Figure 7.4 Excitation order and crosstalk. If the slices are closely spaced, the bases of adjacent slices overlap (crosshatched regions). Tissues located in this overlap region experience RF pulses from both slices and become saturated. This double excitation called crosstalk, causes reduced signal from these regions. The order of slice excitation also determines the contribution of crosstalk to the image intensity. Ascending order of excitation (second row) acquires data from adjacent slice positions in successive time periods. Interleaved ordering (third row) acquires data from every other slice position first, then acquires data from the intermediate positions. This ordering will minimize the effects of crosstalk between all slices.

and contribute little to the detected signal. The slice gap allows space between adjacent slice positions and reduces the extent of crosstalk for the measurement.

Excitation order refers to the temporal order in which slices are excited during the measurement. Two ordering schemes are typically used (see Figure 7.4). Sequential ordering excites adjacent slice positions in successive time periods. This approach is preferred when relative timing of adjacent slices is critical, such as for electrocardiogram-triggered studies of the heart (see Chapter 10). Interleaved ordering excites alternate slices in successive time periods. Interleaved ordering allows the maximum amount of time for $T1$ relaxation of the overlap region prior to the subsequent excitation pulse. The effects of crosstalk are reduced for all slices as much as possible. Arbitrary ordering may also be performed if permitted by the operating software.

The number of partitions, N_{PART}, is used in 3D volume studies and corresponds to the number of slices into which the excited volume is divided. The slices have a signal derived from the total excited volume and are contiguous. The effective slice thickness is the volume excited (thickness) divided by N_{PART}. The scan time for a 3D sequence is linearly proportional to N_{PART} (equation (4.8)).

The field of view, *FOV*, measured in mm², specifies the area from which the MR signals are accurately sampled. The FOV may be specified separately for the readout and phase encoding directions (permitting anisotropic or rectangular FOV) or it may be listed as a single number (isotropic or square FOV). Decreasing the FOV is accomplished by increasing the corresponding gradient amplitude. Increasing spatial resolution may be achieved by decreasing the FOV, which decreases the voxel size at the expense of the SNR.

The acquisition matrix (N_{PE}, N_{RO}) defines the raw data sampling grid used for the measurement of the base image. It consists of two numbers: one specifies the number of phase encoding steps (N_{PE}) and the other specifies the number of readout sampling data points (N_{RO}). Different manufacturers have different conventions regarding which number is specified first. The acquisition matrix divides the FOV into individual areas which, together with the slice thickness, define the voxel size. Increased spatial resolution may be obtained by using larger acquisition matrices to produce smaller voxels. Data acquired beyond that necessary for defining the image FOV is referred to as oversampling and is used to reduce the presence of high-frequency aliasing artifacts (see Chapter 9) and increase the SNR (see Chapter 5). Oversampling in the readout direction does not increase the measurement time, while oversampling in the phase encoding direction increases the scan time proportional to the amount of oversampling.

The number of signal averages, N_{SA} (also known as N_{EX}, the number of excitation pulses), is the number of times the signal from a given slice for a given phase encoding amplitude is measured and added together. Signal averaging is performed in order to increase the SNR ratio. Depending on the operating software, all acquisitions may be performed at each phase encoding amplitude for a slice, or the entire set of phase encoding amplitudes may be measured for each slice before performing the second acquisition for any slice. The SNR is proportional to the square root of N_{SA} while the measurement time is proportional to N_{SA}.

The receiver bandwidth, BW_{REC}, measured in Hz, is the maximum frequency (Nyquist frequency) that can be accurately digitized. The Nyquist frequency depends on the sampling time and N_{RO}. The receiver bandwidth may also be expressed as the total bandwidth over the entire readout FOV or as the bandwidth per pixel (frequency resolution), depending on the particular convention. A lower BW_{REC} improves the SNR at the expense of potentially larger chemical shift artifacts (see Chapter 9).

7.3 Parameter tradeoffs

As mentioned previously, the three criteria used for determining a "good" measurement protocol are sufficient spatial resolution to resolve the underlying anatomy, reasonable signal-difference-to-noise (termed contrast-to-noise) ratio between tissues, and an acceptable measurement time. In general, these three criteria conflict with one another, and the difficulty in protocol optimization is to obtain the proper balance between them. In addition, optimal parameters for one set of tissues may or may not be optimal for another set of tissues. Finally, while each parameter can be specified separately, they are not completely independent. For example, *TE* must be less than *TR*. The following formulas can provide guidance on the tradeoff of one parameter versus another for SNR or image intensity. Tables 7.1 and 7.2 also summarize the parameter changes and their effects on spatial resolution, SNR, and measurement time.

Table 7.1   Measurement effects – extrinsic parameters.

Parameter	Direction of change	Effect on spatial resolution	Effect on S/N ratio	Effect on scan time
TH	Increase	Linear decrease	Linear decrease	None
N_{PART}	Increase	Linear increase	Square root increase	Linear increase
FOV_{RO}	Increase	Linear decrease	Linear decrease	None
FOV_{PE}	Increase	Linear decrease	Linear decrease	None
N_{RO}	Increase	Linear increase	Square root increase	None
N_{PE}	Increase	Linear increase	Square root increase	Linear increase
N_{SA}	Increase	None	Square root increase	Linear increase
BW_{REC}	Increase	None	Square root decrease	None

Table 7.2   Measurement effects – intrinsic parameters.

Parameter	Direction of change	Effect on spatial resolution	Effect on S/N ratio	Effect on scan time
TR	Increase	None	Increase	Linear increase
TE	Increase	None	Decrease	None
Excitation angle, α	Increase	None	Increase for long TR Decrease for short TR	None

7.3.1 Intrinsic variables

Standard single spin echo signal intensity

$$I_{SE} = \exp(-TE/T2) * [1-2 \exp(-[TR-TE/2]/T1) + \exp(-TR/T1)] \tag{7.2}$$

Standard inversion recovery signal intensity

$$I_{IR} = \exp(-TE/T2) * [1 - 2 \exp(-TI/T1) + 2 \exp(-[TR - TE/2]/T1) - \exp(-TR/T1)] \tag{7.3}$$

Standard spoiled gradient echo signal intensity

$$I_{SGE} = \exp(-TE/T2^*) * \sin \alpha * (1 - \exp(-TR/T1))/[1 - \cos \alpha * \exp(-TR/T1)] \tag{7.4}$$

Equations (7.2), (7.3), and (7.4) assume exact RF pulses of the desired excitation angle. For the spin echo and inversion recovery equations, the excitation angle is assumed to be 90° and the refocusing pulses are assumed to be 180°. For the spoiled gradient echo equation, the excitation angle is α.

7.3.2 Extrinsic variables

Standard 2D imaging acquisition

$$SNR_{2D} = R * I * (TH) * (FOV_{RO}/N_{RO}) * (FOV_{PE}/N_{PE}) (N_{SA}N_{RO}N_{PE}/BW_{REC})^{1/2} \qquad (7.5)$$

Standard 3D imaging acquisition

$$SNR_{3D} = R * I * (TH/N_{PART}) * (FOV_{RO}/N_{RO}) * (FOV_{PE}/N_{PE}) * (N_{SA}N_{RO}N_{PE}N_{PART}/BW_{REC})^{1/2}$$

$$(7.6)$$

Equations (7.5) and (7.6) assume uniform tissue content and relaxation behavior throughout the excited volume. R and I contain constants and terms based on the intrinsic parameters as described previously and in equation (5.1). The terms in parentheses represent voxel dimensions and the term inside the square root is the time spent measuring each voxel's signal, so equations 7.5 and 7.6 simplify to equation (5.1). These equations may be used to estimate SNR changes for combinations of parameter changes. For example, the SNR changes in a linear manner with variation in slice thickness, but changes linearly with the square root of N_{SA}; therefore a twofold reduction in slice thickness may be offset by a fourfold increase in N_{SA}.

CHAPTER 8

Signal suppression techniques

Chapter 6 presented the concept of a pulse sequence and described several classes of pulse sequences. The RF and gradient pulses were applied in very precisely defined ways to uniformly affect the signal intensity from all the protons within the volume of measured tissue. Additional RF excitation pulses may be added to any of these sequences to manipulate the net magnetization M of some of the tissue within the imaging volume and differentially affect its contribution to the detected signal. One approach uses frequency-selective saturation pulses, either applied in conjunction with a gradient (spatial presaturation) or in its absence (fat/water saturation, magnetization transfer suppression). Another approach uses the chemical shift frequency difference inherent in tissues to change the relative phase of the signal contribution. This is the basis for water/fat excitation using composite RF pulses and the Dixon method for fat/water suppression. In all of these cases, an increase in the minimal TR for the sequence (sequence kernel time) is required to implement the pulses. In addition, the additional RF pulse(s) increases the total RF power deposition to the patient. Limitations due to the specific rate of RF energy absorption (SAR) (see Chapter 14) may be required, particularly for spin echo-based sequences using short TR.

8.1 Spatial presaturation

 Spatial presaturation pulses are frequency-selective RF pulses applied in conjunction with a gradient pulse based on their location. They have center frequencies and gradient amplitudes different from the pulses used for the imaging volume (Figure 8.1). Spatial presaturation pulses are used to suppress undesired signals from locations within the imaging volume. They are often employed to suppress an artifactual signal from peristaltic and respiratory motion in lumbar spine imaging. They are also used to reduce blood flow artifacts from the aorta or inferior vena cava in abdominal imaging by saturating the blood before it enters the imaging volume. These types of pulses are also used to produce a saturation tag for analyzing the direction of blood flow or cardiac motion.

MRI Basic Principles and Applications, Fifth Edition.
Brian M. Dale, Mark A. Brown and Richard C. Semelka.
© 2015 John Wiley & Sons, Ltd. Published 2015 by John Wiley & Sons, Ltd.

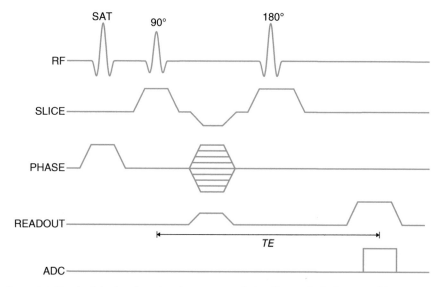

Figure 8.1 Standard single-echo spin echo sequence timing diagram including a spatial presaturation pulse. The saturation pulse (labeled SAT) is applied prior to the primary slice excitation pulse (labeled 90°). The RF pulse center frequency and bandwidth and the gradient amplitudes for the presaturation pulse are independent of these variables for the slice excitation pulses.

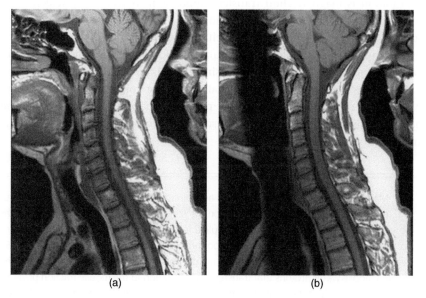

(a)   (b)

Figure 8.2 Application of a spatial presaturation pulse to moving tissue will suppress signal from that tissue. Measurement parameters are: pulse sequence, spin echo; *TR*, 500 ms; *TE*, 16 ms; excitation angle, 90°; acquisition matrix, N_{PE}, 192 and N_{RO}, 256; FOV, 210 mm PE × 280 mm RO; N_{SA}, 3; slice thickness, 4 mm. (a) No presaturation pulse; (b) coronal spatial presaturation pulse, suppressing artifact from swallowing.

Spatial presaturation pulses are usually applied prior to the imaging slice pulses during sequence execution. They may be applied once per slice loop or once per *TR* time period. Due to their rapid occurrence, the presaturation pulses saturate the selected tissue so that its steady-state net magnetization is much smaller than the net magnetization for the remaining tissue of the slice. In addition, spoiler gradients are applied to dephase any residual transverse magnetization following the presaturation pulse. The result is that the signal measured from the presaturated region is significantly less than the signal from the nonpresaturated tissue (Figure 8.2). In addition to the problems regarding sequence kernel times and RF power deposition previously mentioned, spatial presaturation pulses will not remove all signals from the selected region. Tissues in the saturated region experience *T1* relaxation during the time between the presaturation pulse and the imaging excitation pulse so that longitudinal magnetization is present within the presaturated region at the time the slice excitation pulse is applied. This generates a signal from the saturated region that may have significant amplitude, depending on the particular *TR* for the measurement and the tissue *T1* values. The amount of apparent signal suppression depends on the amount of signal produced in the saturated region relative to the signal produced in the unsaturated region.

8.2 Magnetization transfer suppression

Another signal suppression technique similar in implementation to spatial presaturation is magnetization transfer suppression. A frequency-selective RF pulse is used, but in the absence of a gradient, to indirectly saturate tissue water (Figure 8.3). Water within a tissue is either mobile (freely moving) or bound (adsorbed to macromolecules). The bound fraction water protons have a very short *T2* value due to the rapid dephasing they undergo. The resonance peak for these spins is very broad and normally does not contribute significantly to the measured signal. The mobile water molecules have a much longer *T2* and a narrow resonance peak. These two resonances are superimposed at the same center frequency (Figure 8.4).

Magnetization transfer suppression is accomplished using a narrow bandwidth saturation pulse known as a magnetization transfer (MT) pulse centered 1–10 kHz away from the central water frequency applied in the absence of a gradient. Because of their broad resonance peak width, only the bound water protons are irradiated by the RF pulse and become saturated. An exchange occurs between the bound water protons and the unsaturated mobile water protons that transfers the saturation to the mobile fraction protons, causing a loss of steady-state magnetization and reducing the signal from the mobile fraction protons. This process is called magnetization transfer suppression. Contrast is enhanced between tissues that undergo magnetization transfer (water-containing tissues) and those that do not (fat-containing tissues). Magnetization transfer pulses are used in spin echo or gradient echo sequences to produce additional signal suppression of tissue water.

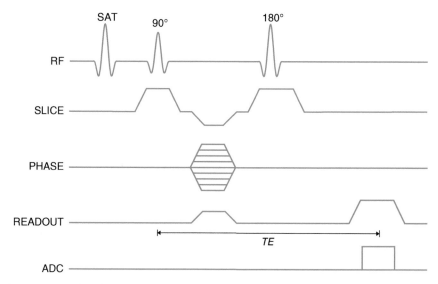

Figure 8.3 Standard single-echo spin echo sequence timing diagram, including a frequency-selective presaturation pulse. The saturation pulse (labeled SAT) is applied prior to the primary slice excitation pulse (labeled 90°). The RF pulse center frequency and bandwidth for the presaturation pulse are independent of these variables for the slice excitation pulses. Note the absence of the associated gradient pulse for the presaturation pulse compared to Figure 8.1.

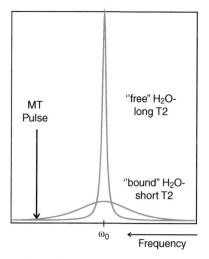

Figure 8.4 Magnetization transfer suppression. Mobile or "free" tissue water has protons with long $T2$ values and produces a narrow resonance peak. Water adsorbed or "bound" to macromolecules has protons with short $T2$ values and produces a wide resonance peak normally not visualized in an image. Both types of water protons have the same resonant frequency. The magnetization transfer RF pulse is applied at a frequency different (off-resonance) from the water to saturate the bound water protons. Exchange between the bound and free water transfers the saturation to the free water protons, reducing signal intensity from the free water.

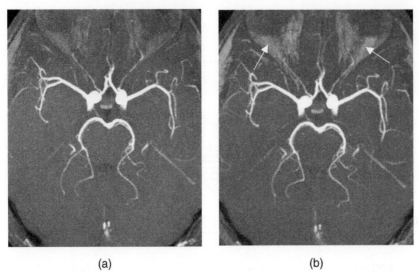

(a)   (b)

Figure 8.5 Effects of magnetization transfer in three-dimensional MR angiography. Application of MT pulse suppressed background signal from gray and white matter, enabling better visualization of blood vessels. An apparent increase in signal from suborbital fat is observed (arrows). Measurement parameters are: pulse sequence, three-dimensional refocused gradient echo, postexcitation; TR, 42 ms; TE, 7 ms; excitation angle, 25°; acquisition matrix, N_{PE}, 192 and N_{RO} 512 with twofold readout oversampling; FOV, 201 mm PE × 230 mm RO; N_{SA}, 1; effective slice thickness, 0.78 mm. (a) No MT pulse; (b) MT pulse.

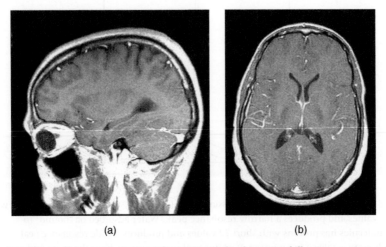

(a)   (b)

Figure 8.6 Effects of magnetization transfer in $T1$-weighted imaging following contrast administration. Application of MT pulse suppresses background signal from normal matter, enabling better visualization of contrast-enhanced tissues such as tumors or vascular structures. (a) No MT pulse; (b) MT pulse.

Magnetization transfer suppression is most often used to reduce a signal from normal tissue water in studies where this tissue is of little interest. Two examples illustrate this. Time-of-flight MR angiography (see Chapter 11) is a technique for visualizing blood flow within the vascular network. Suppression of the normal brain tissue water using magnetization transfer pulses enables smaller vessels to be distinguished (Figure 8.5). The other application of magnetization transfer is *T1* studies following the administration of a contrast agent. *T1* contrast agents shorten the *T1* relaxation time for tissues where the agent is located (see Chapter 15). Comparison of images acquired before and after contrast administration enables determination of the agent dispersal within a tissue. Use of a magnetization transfer pulse during the postcontrast measurement reduces the signal from the unenhanced tissues, increasing their contrast with the enhanced tissue (Figure 8.6).

8.3 Frequency-selective saturation

Another application for a frequency-selective saturation pulse without an accompanying gradient is to directly suppress signals from spins that are visualized in an image. The spins that are typically selected are either fat or water protons. Normal MR imaging methods visualize protons from both water and fat molecules within the tissue. As mentioned in Chapter 2, fat and water have a chemical shift difference of approximately 3.5 ppm to their resonant frequencies. Frequency-selective saturation uses a narrow bandwidth RF pulse centered at either the fat or water resonant frequency applied in the absence of a gradient (Figure 8.7). The resulting transverse magnetization is then dephased by spoiler gradients. A standard imaging sequence may then be performed, which produces images from the

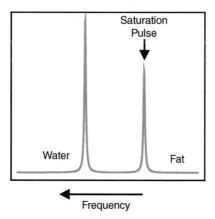

Frequency

Figure 8.7 Frequency spectrum of fat and water. Fat saturation applies an additional RF excitation pulse centered at the fat resonant frequency. This pulse is applied prior to the primary slice excitation pulse, so that the signal from the slice is produced primarily from the water.

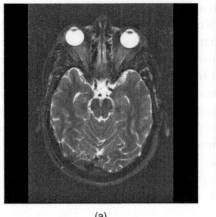 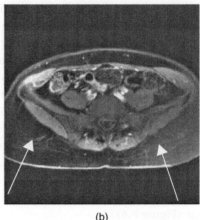

(a)   (b)

Figure 8.8 Frequency-selective saturation (fatsat) pulse is applied to suppress signal from fat protons. (a) With a homogeneous magnetic field, the suppression of fat is uniform throughout the slice; (b) with a nonhomogeneous magnetic field, the saturation pulse suppresses fat well in one region of the image and poorly in another region (arrows).

other type of protons within the slice (Figure 8.8a). The number of saturation pulses applied during the sequence loop is variable, ranging from once per *TR* time period to once per slice excitation pulse. The signal suppression mechanism is similar to that of spatial presaturation described previously, in that minimal net magnetization from the saturated protons is present at the time of the excitation pulse for the slice.

While signal from either fat or water protons may be suppressed using frequency-selective presaturation, its most frequent usage is for suppression of fat. Fat saturation has two main advantages over STIR imaging (see Chapter 6) for fat suppression. It may be incorporated into virtually any type of imaging sequence. *T1* fat saturation sequences may also be used with gadolinium-based *T1* contrast agents since the contrast agent shortens the *T1* relaxation times of only the water protons (see Chapter 15). The *T1* reduction enables the enhanced tissues to generate significant signal while the fat signal remains minimal in the presence or absence of the contrast agent.

Three potential problems are inherent with frequency-selective presaturation, in addition to the problems of increased slice loop time and RF power deposition. One is that there will be magnetization transfer suppression (see above) of the water protons by the saturation pulse if fat saturation is performed. The second problem is that the saturated protons undergo *T1* relaxation during the time between the saturation pulse and the imaging pulses and will contribute to the detected signal. Multiple fat saturation pulses within a slice loop may be necessary to achieve the desired signal suppression, increasing the required *TR*.

Finally, frequency-selective presaturation is particularly sensitive to the magnetic field homogeneity. The exact resonant frequency for a fat and a water proton depend upon the magnetic field that a voxel experiences. If the homogeneity is not uniform throughout the imaging volume, the center frequency of the saturation pulse will be off-resonance for some of the spins and will not be effective in suppression (Figure 8.8b). In some cases, the water protons may be saturated rather than the fat protons. For this reason, optimization of the field homogeneity to the specific patient prior to applying a frequency-selective presaturation pulse is advisable.

8.4 Nonsaturation methods

Two methods for signal suppression rely on the inherent frequency difference between fat and water, but are not saturation-based techniques. One method uses a gradient echo sequence with a composite RF pulse (see Chapter 5) for slice/volume excitation. Known as water excitation, the pulse amplitudes and relative timings within the composite pulse are chosen to selectively excite the water protons and leave the fat protons unexcited (Figure 8.9). Composite pulses are very sensitive to field homogeneity since differences in the resonant frequency change the cycling time for fat relative to water. Poor homogeneity causes undesired excitation and/or incomplete suppression. For this reason, optimization of the field homogeneity to each patient is advisable.

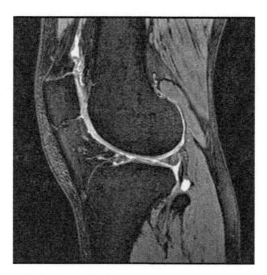

Figure 8.9 Water excitation image acquired using a composite RF pulse. Measurement parameters:pulse sequence, three-dimensional gradient echo, combination pre-and postexcitation; TR, 25.4 ms; TE, 9 ms; excitation angle, 35° cumulative; acquisition matrix, N_{PE}, 256 and N_{RO}, 256; FOV, 160 mm PE × 160 mm RO; N_{SA}, 1; effective slice thickness, 1.56 mm.

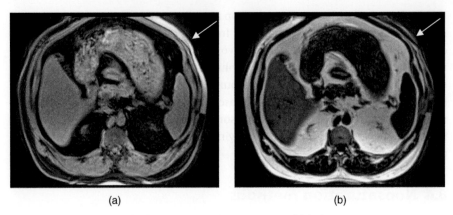

Figure 8.10 Dixon method for fat suppression: (a) water image; (b) fat image. Poor magnet homogeneity results in a phase wrap, causing the fat and water to appear in the incorrect images (arrows).

Another method for fat suppression is known as the Dixon method (Dixon, 1984), which is a mathematical model-based approach and can be used both with spin echo and gradient echo scans. Recall in Chapter 6 that the spin echo pulse sequence has both an RF echo and a gradient echo that are superimposed in time during signal collection. The resulting image will have both fat and water contributing with the same signal phase. If the gradient prephase area in the readout direction is modified, then the fat echo can be made to be 180° in phase relative to the spin echo. This will reverse the relative fat contribution in the detected signal. Addition of the two images will create an image of only water, while subtraction will create an image of only fat (Figure 8.10). Subsequent refinements have made the Dixon method very insensitive to field homogeneity by accounting for differences in the resonant frequency that change the cycling time for fat relative to water. Acquisition of a third echo with a different amount of fat contribution may be necessary to avoid artifacts such as illustrated in Figure 8.10.

CHAPTER 9

Artifacts

 Artifacts in MR images refer to pixels that do not faithfully represent the anatomy being studied. In the images, the general appearance is that the underlying anatomy is visualized but spurious signals are present that do not correspond to actual tissue at that location. The artifacts may or may not be easily discernible from normal anatomy, particularly if they are of low intensity, and may or may not be reproducible. Artifacts can be categorized in many ways. One approach divides them into three groups, according to the cause of the signal misregistration. The first group is a consequence of motion of patient tissue during the measurement. This includes both gross physical motion by the patient and internal physiological motion such as blood flow. The second group is produced primarily as a result of the particular measurement technique and/or specific measurement parameters. The final group of artifacts are independent of the patient or measurement technique, being generated either through a malfunction of the MR scanner during data collection or from a source external to the patient or scanner.

9.1 Motion artifacts

Motion artifacts occur as a result of movement of tissue during the data acquisition period. They are manifest as signal misregistrations in the phase encoding direction, though the specific appearance of the artifact depends on the nature of the motion and the particular measurement technique. The artifacts are caused by tissue that is excited at one location, producing signals that are mapped to a different location during detection. As mentioned in Chapter 4, the typical MRI scan excites and detects a signal from a tissue volume multiple times with the phase encoding gradient G_{PE} changing amplitude prior to signal detection. The assumption is made that any measured signal intensity variations from one measurement to the next are as a result of G_{PE} only. When tissue moves, the protons are at a different location at the time of detection and experience a different G_{RO} amplitude, contributing a different frequency and phase for that measurement. The Fourier transformation mismaps these protons to an incorrect location along the phase encoding direction in the image. The misregistered signals occur along the phase encoding direction rather than the readout direction because G_{RO} is identical for each signal that is measured, while G_{PE} changes from line to line. In addition, the encoding

MRI Basic Principles and Applications, Fifth Edition.
Brian M. Dale, Mark A. Brown and Richard C. Semelka.
© 2015 John Wiley & Sons, Ltd. Published 2015 by John Wiley & Sons, Ltd.

of phase by G_{PE} occurs prior to signal detection while it occurs concurrent with signal detection for G_{RO}. In general, many measurements are made in the production of an image, each with a different amount of motion contamination.

The sensitivity of a measurement to tissue motion depends on the amount of frequency and phase variation that occurs between successive echoes due to the tissue movement. If the motion occurs during measurements with high positive or negative G_{PE} (at the edges of k-space), then the misregistered signal will have very little amplitude and will generate minimal artifact regardless of the nature of the motion. If the motion occurs during measurements with low amplitude G_{PE} (low magnitude k_y), the nature of the motion and the measurement technique will affect the artifact appearance. If the echo timing is relatively slow or the motion is at a moderate rate, significant artifact will be generated since there will be significant signal measured from different locations. If the time between successive echoes (echo spacing in echo train sequences, TR for traditional sequences) is rapid and the motion is relatively slow, the echoes near the center of k-space may be acquired with the tissue in the same location, so that there is minimal artifactual signal generated. This is the principle behind the use of single-shot ETSE for visualizing the small bowel.

The artifact appearance also depends on the nature of the motion. If the motion itself is periodic, then the misregistration artifacts will be discrete in nature, often referred to as "ghosts". The "ghost" signals will offset in the phase encoding direction from the primary anatomy at locations inversely proportional to the difference between the period of the motion and the TR of the scan. The sequence looping may also affect which images of the scan will show motion artifacts, subject to the G_{PE} discussion above. For scans with one subloop, all images will generally exhibit motion artifacts. For scans with multiple subloops, artifacts will be present for all images within a subloop where the motion occurs. When interleaved acquisition ordering is used, images at adjacent slice positions may show different amounts of artifact contamination.

Probably the most common motion artifact in MRI is due to blood flow. The artifact from blood flow is dependent on the nature of the flow and its direction relative to the slice orientation. Through-plane flow (flow that is perpendicular to the slice plane) typically produces a localized artifact in the image with a width equal to the vessel diameter and in line with the source of the flow. Flow that is relatively fast compared to TR will produce a relatively continuous artifact throughout the FOV, such as in spin echo images (Figure 9.1a). Flow that is slow relative to TR may not generate an artifact as significant saturation will occur unless a contrast agent is used to shorten the $T1$ relaxation time of the blood. If the flow is relatively periodic such as pulsatile flow, then the artifact appears as "ghost" vessels at discrete intervals. This is often seen from blood flow in the aorta or inferior vena cava (IVC) in transverse slices of the abdomen acquired with gradient echo images (Figure 9.1b). In-plane flow (flow that is parallel to the slice plane) produces a more diffuse artifact, which can be observed from the aorta and IVC in coronal images. The vessel extends through the entire image field and thus the artifact affects all regions of the image (Figure 9.2a). Flow of the cerebrospinal fluid in the brain and spinal canal are also problematic and can produce analogous artifacts on $T2$-weighted images (Figure 9.2b).

In abdominal or lumbar spine imaging, respiratory motion and peristalsis are the most common causes of a severe artifactual signal. The movement of the abdomen during the data collection process produces multiple misregistration artifacts. If the respiration rate is constant, the "ghost" images are either few in number or discrete and offset in the phase encoding direction from the true image by an amount proportional to the respiration rate.

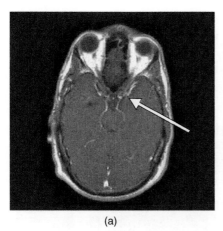 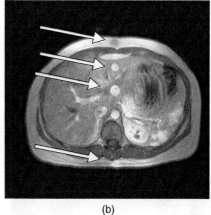

(a) (b)

Figure 9.1 Flow misregistration artifact, through-plane. (a) Flow fast compared to measurement technique produces "zipper"-like artifact (arrow). Measurement technique: pulse sequence, spin echo; *TR*, 479 ms; *TE*, 17 ms; acquisition matrix, N_{PE}, 192 and N_{RO} 256; FOV, 172 mm PE × 230 mm RO; N_{SA}, 1; slice thickness, 5 mm. PE direction: R–L; RO direction: A–P. (b) Periodic flow from the aorta will be misregistered as multiple ghosts (arrows). Measurement parameters are: pulse sequence, two-dimensional spoiled gradient echo; *TR*, 164 ms; *TE*, 4 ms; excitation angle, 70°; acquisition matrix, N_{PE}, 134 and N_{RO} 256; FOV, 262 mm PE × 350 mm RO; N_{SA}, 1; slice thickness, 5 mm; PE direction, A–P; RO direction, L–R.

If the respiration rate is variable, the "ghost" images are numerous and appear as a smearing of signal throughout the entire image (Figure 9.3a). For segmented techniques such as echo train spin echo techniques, respiratory motion may appear as multiple lines or so-called "venetian blinds" superimposed throughout the entire FOV in the phase encoding direction. The number and spacing of the lines is based on the number of segments for the scan (Figure 9.3b). Peristalsis produces motion artifacts that are less distinct than those from respiratory motion. In most instances, a general blurring of the large and small bowel occurs and a layer of noise is superimposed over the entire image.

9.2 Sequence/Protocol-related artifacts

A second class of artifacts results from the specific measurement process used to acquire the image. While the appearance of motion artifacts also depends on the particular measurement protocol, this group of artifacts is more sensitive to technical aspects of the particular pulse sequence and method of data collection used. The source of these artifacts is relatively constant over the course of the measurement and the resulting signal misregistrations are easily recognized when present.

9.2.1 Aliasing
The techniques used for spatial localization assign a unique frequency and phase to each location within the image. These are determined by the acquisition matrix and the desired FOV

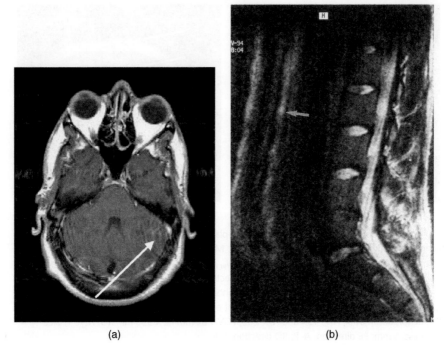

(a)   (b)

Figure 9.2 Flow misregistration artifact, in-plane. (a) In-plane blood flow will produce severe signal misregistration (arrow). Measurement technique: pulse sequence, spin echo; TR, 479 ms; TE, 17 ms; acquisition matrix, N_{PE}, 192 and N_{RO}, 256; FOV, 172 mm PE × 230 mm RO; N_{SA}, 1; slice thickness, 5 mm; PE direction: R–L; RO direction: A–P. (b) Flow misregistration artifact. Flowing CSF will be misregistered as a ghost canal (arrow). Measurement parameters are: pulse sequence, spin echo; TR, 2500 ms; TE, 90 ms; excitation angle, 90°; acquisition matrix, N_{PE}, 192 and N_{RO}, 256 with twofold frequency oversampling; FOV, 210 mm PE × 280 mm RO; N_{SA}, 1; slice thickness, 5 mm; PE direction, A–P; RO direction, H–R.

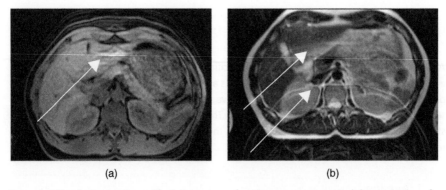

(a)   (b)

Figure 9.3 Respiratory motion artifact. Extraneous ghost images are generated due to motion of the abdominal wall during data acquisition (arrows). The number and severity of the ghosts depends on the TR, respiration rate, and the particular measurement technique. (a) Pulse sequence, two-dimensional spoiled gradient echo; TR, 159 ms; (b) pulse sequence, echo train spin echo; TR, 4000 ms.

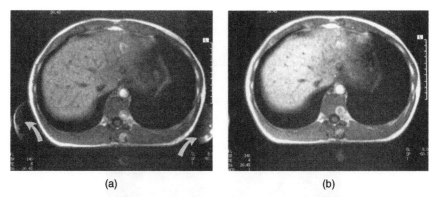

(a)   (b)

Figure 9.4 Effects of oversampling. (a) Without frequency oversampling, frequencies for the protons within the arms exceed the Nyquist limit and are aliased or incorrectly mapped into the image (arrows). Measurement parameters are: pulse sequence, two-dimensional spoiled gradient echo; TR, 140 ms; TE, 4 ms; excitation angle, 80°; acquisition matrix, N_{PE}, 128 and N_{RO}, 256; FOV, 263 mm PE × 350 mm RO; N_{SA}, 1; slice thickness, 8 mm. (b) Same as (a) except with frequency oversampling. The frequencies for the protons within the arms are measured accurately by increasing the number of readout data points measured during the same sampling time while maintaining the same G_{RO}. Only frequencies corresponding to the FOV selected are stored so that the arms are excluded from the final image. Measurement parameters are the same as (a), except that $N_{RO} = 512$.

in the phase-encoding and readout directions. Aliasing in the readout direction occurs when tissue outside the chosen FOV_{RO} is excited. This can occur if an FOV_{RO} smaller than the anatomical slice is selected. The frequencies for this tissue exceed the Nyquist limit for the sampling conditions and are mapped to a lower frequency, a situation known as high-frequency aliasing or frequency wraparound (Figure 9.4a). The technique used to overcome this is known as frequency oversampling, in which the dwell time per point is reduced by increasing the number of readout data points while maintaining the same sampling time. The same G_{RO} is used, which results in an increase in the span of k_x using the same Δk. The oversampled data results in an increase of the Nyquist frequency ω_{NQ} for the measurement, according to equation (2.2). Because G_{RO} is constant, the frequencies at the chosen FOV_{RO} are unchanged, so that extraction of the central range of frequencies produces an image of the desired size and number of data points. For example, for a 256 × 256 matrix with twofold frequency oversampling, 512 data points are measured but only the central 256 data points are used to create the image (Figure 9.4b).

Aliasing can also occur in the phase encoding direction when tissue outside the FOV_{PE} are excited. The protons within this region undergo phase changes corresponding to frequencies greater than can be accurately measured for the G_{PE} pulse duration (Nyquist limit). They are mapped via the Fourier transformation to a lower phase, in a manner analogous to the aliasing in the readout direction described above. Phase encoding aliasing can only be eliminated by increasing the effective FOV_{PE} for the scan. This may be accomplished either by reducing the change in gradient amplitude Δk_y from one phase encoding step to the next (increasing the FOV_{PE}) or by increasing the number of phase changes (i.e., Nyquist frequency) while maintaining the same Δk_y, a technique known as phase encoding oversampling. Because more echoes are acquired, phase encoding oversampling will increase the total measurement time while also improving the SNR.

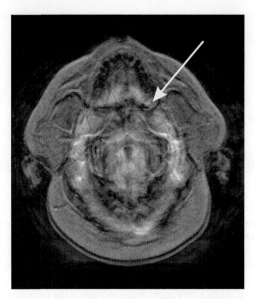

Figure 9.5 Three-dimensional volume scan showing high-frequency aliasing in the slice-selection direction. The superior part of the brain (arrow) appears in the inferior slices of the imaging volume.

Aliasing can also occur in the slice-selection direction in 3D scanning in certain situations. The excitation pulse must be nonselective and the k_z volume spanned by the 3D encoding table must be smaller than the volume of tissue excited. In this case, anatomy from slices at one edge of the volume will wrap into the opposite side of the volume (Figure 9.5). Similar to the case of aliasing in the phase-encoding direction, the remedy for aliasing in the slice direction is to increase the effective area of accurate measurement, either though increased Δk_z (increasing the effective slice thickness) or through slice oversampling (more k_z samples with constant Δk_z).

Parallel acquisition techniques can also show aliasing artifacts. As mentioned in Chapter 5, the measurement process uses larger Δk_y values compared to a conventional scan. As a result, the effective FOV_{PE} for a coil is smaller, so that aliasing occurs for the signal in each coil. If the image-based techniques are used, this aliasing is indistinguishable from aliasing produced if the base FOV_{PE} is too small for the anatomy under observation. This causes more severe aliasing artifacts than for the conventional scan (Figure 9.6a). Phase oversampling could be incorporated in the scan protocol, but this would increase the scan time. Increasing the base FOV_{PE} is the best option to eliminate the additional artifact. In contrast, the k-space-based techniques will generate more diffuse artifacts, with no additional aliasing artifacts (Figure 9.6b).

9.2.2 Chemical shift artifacts

Chemical shift-based artifacts arise from the inherent 3.5 ppm frequency difference between fat and water protons under the influence of an external magnetic field as described in Chapter 2. Two constant artifacts may be generated by this frequency difference. One is known as the chemical shift artifact, which is a misregistration of fat and water protons from a voxel that are mapped to different pixels. As described in Chapter 4, the detected signal from a voxel

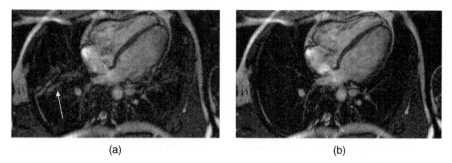

(a)   (b)

Figure 9.6 Small FOV aliasing artifacts with parallel acquisitions: (a) image-based parallel acquisition; (b) *k*-space-based acquisition. Note the aliasing artifact in the lung field in (a) (arrow) due to the anatomical region being larger than the scan FOV. This area is artifact-free in (b).

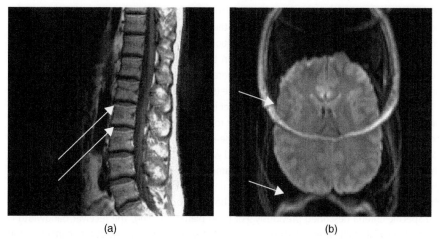

(a)   (b)

Figure 9.7 Chemical shift artifact. (a) Note alternate bands of light and dark at the interface between the vertebrae and disk (arrows). Measurement parameters: pulse sequence, spin echo; Receiver bandwidth, 20 kHz; readout direction, H–F. (b) A complete misregistration of fat from the bone marrow of the skull (arrow). Measurement parameters are: pulse sequence, spin echo EPI; phase-encoding direction, A–P.

is mapped to a position based on its frequency according to equation (4.1), under the assumption that all protons within a voxel resonate at the same frequency. Due to the difference in molecular structure, fat protons have an intrinsically lower resonant frequency than water protons when exposed to the same external magnetic field. Fat protons within a voxel are affected by the same G_{RO} as the water protons but will be mapped to a lower frequency pixel in the readout direction. This frequency misregistration is not noticeable in tissues with a uniform fat–water content, but can be seen at the borders between tissues with a significantly different fat–water content; for example, between a disk and vertebrae in the spine or between the kidney and retroperitoneal fat. Parallel areas of bright and dark pixels can be visualized where the fat and water signals superimpose and where they do not, respectively (Figure 9.7a). The number of pixels corresponding to the chemical shift artifact (CSA) depends upon the frequency difference in Hz between fat and water, the total receiver bandwidth, and the number of readout data points spanning the FOV_{RO}:

$$CSA = \Delta\omega * N_{RO}/BW_{REC} \qquad\qquad (9.1)$$

At 1.5 T, the frequency difference, $\Delta\omega$, is approximately 220 Hz so that, for a scan with a total receiver bandwidth of 20 kHz and $N_{RO} = 256$, the CSA will be 2.8 pixels. The severity of the artifact in the final image will depend on the FOV_{RO}. If an FOV_{RO} of 350 mm is used, this translates into a fat/water misregistration of 3.6 mm. For an FOV_{RO} of 175 mm, the artifact is only 1.8 mm. For a scan with a receiver bandwidth of 33 kHz, the CSA will be 1.7 pixels and a misregistration of 2.2 mm. Chemical shift artifacts are most prominent at magnetic field strengths greater than 1.5 T, using low or narrow receiver bandwidths and large FOV_{RO}, and at fat–water tissue interfaces. For example, at 3 T, the same 33 kHz receiver bandwidth and 256 readout points will produce a CSA of 3.4 pixels.

In theory, chemical shift artifacts are possible in all three directions (slice selection, phase encoding, and readout), since magnetic field variations (gradient pulses) are used for localization in all cases. In the slice selection direction, the RF pulse bandwidth and gradient amplitude are chosen to keep this at a minimum. In addition, because the slice selection direction is not directly visualized, any signal misregistration in this direction is difficult to discern. This may not be the case in MR spectroscopic scans, where there may be observable variations in signal amplitude at different locations within the slice (see Chapter 13).

The appearance of the chemical shift artifact in the readout and phase encoding directions depends on the particular pulse sequence. For routine imaging techniques such as spin echo, echo train spin echo, or gradient echo, the phase-encoding process is reinitiated following each excitation pulse. Since Δk_y is constant, fat and water protons located at the same position in the phase encoding direction undergo equal amounts of phase change. They are mapped to the same location in the image in the phase encoding direction and no artifact results. For these techniques, chemical shift artifacts may be observed in the readout direction, based on the specific criteria described previously. For echo planar imaging, the receiver bandwidth is normally very large (in excess of 100 kHz) so that fat and water frequencies are mapped to the same pixel. However, the phase encoding process for the entire image occurs in a continuous fashion following one or two excitation pulses. Chemical shift artifacts are observed in the phase-encoding direction and are very significant. Because the G_{PE} amplitude is very low, the misregistration may be as much as 12–15 pixels (Figure 9.7b). Use of fat suppression techniques is necessary to minimize the artifact.

9.2.3 Phase cancellation artifact

The second artifact induced by the chemical shift difference is known as the phase cancellation artifact (or sometimes the chemical shift artifact of the second kind), observed in out-of-phase gradient echo images. As shown in Figure 2.6, the fat protons cycle in phase relative to the water proton precession at a rate linearly proportional to the measurement time after the initial RF excitation pulse. For normal spin echo and fast spin echo sequences, this phase cycling is exactly reversed by the 180° RF pulse(s) so that the fat and water protons always contribute to the signal at the echo time, TE, with the same polarity; that is, the fat and water protons are described as "in phase" when the signal is detected regardless of the choice of TE. This assumes that the 180° RF pulse occurs halfway between the initial RF excitation pulse and TE. In gradient echo sequences, the phase cycling is not reversed (since there is no 180° RF pulse)

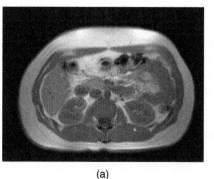 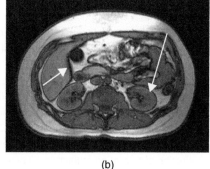

(a)   (b)

Figure 9.8 Phase cancellation artifact. Other measurement parameters are: pulse sequence, two-dimensional spoiled gradient echo; TR, 164 ms; excitation angle, 70°; acquisition matrix, N_{PE}, 134 and N_{RO}, 256; FOV, 263 mm PE × 350 mm RO; N_{SA}, 1; slice thickness, 9 mm. (a) In-phase image (TE, 4.5 ms). Fat and water protons have the same phase and contribute in the same fashion to the image contrast. (b) Out-of-phase image (TE, 2.2 ms). Fat and water protons have opposite phases and contribute in opposite fashion to the image contrast. For voxels with equal amounts of fat and water, such as at the interface between liver or kidney and retroperitoneal fat, cancellation of signal occurs, producing a dark band (arrows).

so that fat and water protons contribute differently to the detected signal, depending on the particular TE. Voxels containing both fat and water have additional signal intensity variations in addition to those due to relaxation. For certain choices of TE, known as "out-of-phase" TE, very little signal is produced if the voxel has equal water and fat content, such as those voxels located at interfaces between fat- and water-based tissues. This signal cancellation appears as a dark ring surrounding the tissue (Figure 9.8).

The TE values that generate this phase cancellation depend on the magnetic field strength, since the time for the phase cycling depends upon the resonant frequency difference, $\Delta\omega$ in Hz, between fat and water:

$$TE_{\text{in-phase}} = n/\Delta\omega \tag{9.2}$$

where n is an integer. The out-of-phase TE times occur midway between the in-phase times (Table 9.1). Out-of-phase images are often used to assess the amount of fat contribution to a voxel. The phase cancellation artifact observed using out-of-phase TE makes it difficult to assess the interface of tissues with different fat and water content. The phase cycling also affects the signal content of all tissues throughout the image.

Table 9.1 Phase cycling TE times.

Field strength, T	In-phase TE, ms	Out-of-phase TE, ms
0.5	13.3, 26.67	6.67, 20
1.0	6.67, 13.3, 20	3.3, 10, 16.67
1.5	4.5, 9.0, 13.5, 18.0	2.25, 6.75, 11.25, 15.75
3.0	2.25, 4.5, 6.75, 9.0	1.12, 3.38, 5.63, 7.88

9.2.4 Truncation artifacts

Truncation artifacts are produced by insufficient digital sampling of the echo. The most common instance of this condition occurs when data collection is terminated while significant signal is still being induced in the receiver coil by the protons; for example, in T1-weighted imaging where there is a high signal from fat still present at the end of data collection. The Fourier transformation of this truncated data set produces a "ringing" type of signal oscillation that emanates from the edge of the anatomy (Figure 9.9). Truncation artifacts can also occur if the echo is sampled in an asymmetrical fashion; that is, the echo is not sampled equally on both sides of the echo maximum (Figure 9.10). This type of data sampling is often used in very short TE sequences (<3 ms) to minimize the receiver bandwidth.

Reduction of truncation artifacts involves reducing the signal amplitude so that it is minimal at the beginning or end of the data collection period. This reduction can be achieved in two ways. One approach is to reduce the fat signal through fat suppression (since fat typically has the largest signal in T1-weighted images), either using a fat saturation pulse or using an inversion recovery technique with an appropriate TI time. This approach changes the intrinsic image contrast and may be unacceptable for the particular clinical application. The other method is to apply an apodization filter to the raw data prior to Fourier transformation. This numerical process forces the signal amplitude to zero at the end of the data collection period. Several types of apodization filters have been developed (e.g., Fermi, Gaussian, Hanning), each with different characteristics regarding the filter shape (Figure 9.11). Use of apodization filters improves the signal-to-noise ratio by removing high-frequency noise from the signal. However, excessive filtering eliminates high frequencies responsible for fine spatial resolution or edge definition so that blurring is possible. Asymmetric echo sampling may require more extensive filtering to reduce truncation artifacts. Acquiring the echo in a symmetric fashion reduces the amount of filtering necessary.

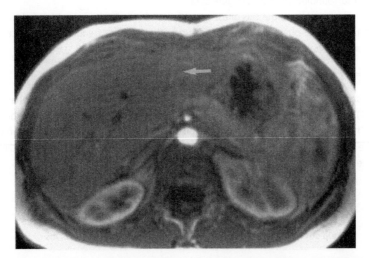

Figure 9.9 Truncation artifact. Image acquisition with asymmetric sampling produces a banding artifact (arrow), originating from the high signal of subcutaneous fat. Measurement parameters: pulse sequence, two-dimensional spoiled gradient echo; TR, 170 ms; TE, 4 ms; excitation angle, 80°; acquisition matrix, N_{PE}, 144 and N_{RO}, 256 with twofold oversampling; FOV, 262 mm PE × 350 mm RO; N_{SA}, 1.

TE   TE

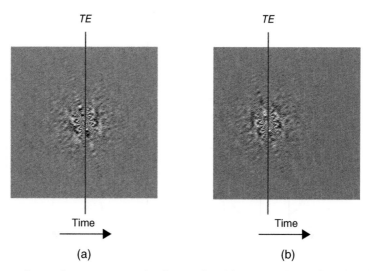

Time   Time

(a)   (b)

Figure 9.10 Symmetric versus asymmetric echo sampling. (a) In symmetric sampling, the echo is maximum (*TE*) midway through the sampling period, so that both sides of the echo signal are measured equally. Filtering of the data can be performed in a symmetrical fashion. (b) In asymmetric sampling, the echo maximum is in the early portion of the sampling period. Significant signal is present when the sampling begins and filtering of the signal is difficult.

9.2.5 Coherence artifacts

Coherence artifacts are a class of artifacts that can have a variable appearance, based on the particular measurement technique and how it is implemented on the scanner. They are produced by the RF pulses generating unwanted transverse magnetization that contributes to the detected signal. One coherence artifact is known as an FID artifact. As mentioned in Chapter 4, the RF excitation pulses are not uniform in profile. For instance, while most of the protons in a slice would experience a 180° excitation pulse, those located at the edges of the slice would experience a range of excitation angles, all less than 180°. The FID produced by these protons may still have significant amplitude when the desired echo signal is measured. Because the 180° RF pulse normally occurs after the phase encoding gradient during sequence execution, the induced signal will contribute identically during each ADC sampling period. The resulting artifact is a line of constant phase in the final image that is superimposed on the line of zero phase (Figure 9.12).

Another coherence artifact may be produced by the effects of the multiple RF excitation pulses on the protons. The spin echoes used to produce *T1*- and *T2*-weighted images are but two of several echoes generated by RF excitation pulses within an imaging sequence. For example, a series of three RF pulses such as a presaturation pulse and a 90–180° pulse pair or a 90–180–180° pulse trio may generate four or five echoes. The timing and number of echoes depends on the exact spacing of the pulses (Figure 9.13). The amplitude of each echo depends on the excitation angle of the individual pulses and the particular tissues being measured. These "secondary" echoes contain all the frequency information of the so-called primary echoes normally used, but have different *T1* and *T2* weighting to the signals. Should these other echoes occur while the ADC is sampling the primary echoes, they will contribute to the final image. These "extra" echoes may produce either line artifacts if not phase encoded or an

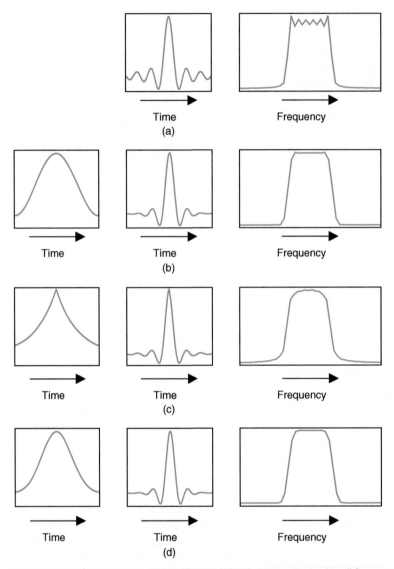

Figure 9.11 Raw data filtering. All vertical and horizontal scales are maintained in all figures. (a) Unfiltered sinc pulse waveform, time domain (left) and magnitude frequency domain (right) (note sawtooth pattern at top of right figure); (b) Gaussian filter (left), Gaussian-filtered sinc pulse waveform, time domain (center) and magnitude frequency domain (right). (note that sawtooth pattern at top of right figure is reduced but still present); (c) Fermi filter (left), Fermi-filtered sinc pulse waveform, time domain (center) and magnitude frequency domain (right) (note rounded top and large width at base of right figure); (d) Hanning filter (left), Hanning-filtered sinc pulse waveform, time domain (center) and magnitude frequency domain (right).

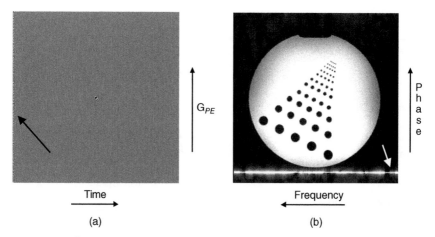

G_{PE}

Time

Frequency

P
h
a
s
e

(a)   (b)

Figure 9.12 Insufficient spoiling, raw data and image. Due to the imperfect nature of RF pulses, additional signal can be produced by spins at the edge of the slice. If the spurious signal is generated by the 180° pulse in a spin echo pulse sequence, it is not affected by the phase encoding process and appears as a constant signal in k-space (arrow in a). The resulting image shows a bright line near the edge of the image FOV (arrow in b).

additional image if phase encoded (Figure 9.14). One of these echoes, known as the stimulated echo, is incorporated into the design of fast spin echo imaging techniques and in the volume selection process used in MR spectroscopy (Chapter 13).

Pulse sequences are usually designed with great care to minimize the contamination of the desired echo signals by the undesired echoes. When these undesired echoes form during the ADC sampling period due to the particular RF pulse timing, some form of coherence "spoiling" is used. Two approaches are used to minimize the coherence present from these secondary echoes during sampling. The most common method is to include additional gradient pulses applied at appropriate times during the pulse sequence, an approach known as gradient spoiling. The goal is to change the time when the coherence forms so that it occurs when the ADC is not sampling. These gradient pulses are usually of high amplitude and/or long duration. The time when these pulses are applied depends on which coherence is to be spoiled and what TE is chosen. Spoiler gradients applied following the 180° refocusing pulse reduce the FID artifact resulting from nonuniform RF excitation. Spoiler gradients following the data collection such as those used in spin echo sequences (see Figure 6.2) minimizes coherence contamination of the subsequent echoes. Gradient spoiling may also use a series of amplitudes rather than a constant amplitude pulse in order to improve spoiling if the RF interpulse time is short.

If the TR is short compared to the tissue $T2$, as is frequently used in gradient echo scanning, then significant coherence artifacts can occur from the standard RF excitation pulses. Use of gradient spoiling requires gradient pulse durations that can be 30–50% of the slice loop. For spoiled gradient echo sequences, another approach for spoiling is frequently used, known as RF spoiling. Normal data acquisition techniques apply RF pulses of constant phase or with a 180° phase alternation of the excitation pulse (i.e., +90°, –90°, +90°, …). The receiver is also phase-alternated to match the transmitter phase so that signal averaging can be performed. RF spoiling applies a phase variation other than ±90° or ±180° to the excitation pulse and receiver. The desired echo signals add in a coherent fashion, while the other

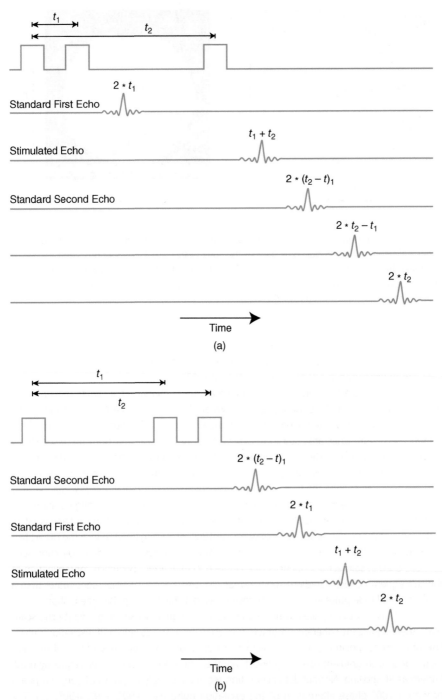

Figure 9.13 Echo timing plots. (a) Time t_1 is less than t_2, typical of a standard short *TE* / long *TE* spin echo pulse sequence. Five echoes are formed. Two are used in routine imaging (echoes 1 and 3). The stimulated echo occurs at time $t_1 + t_2$ (echo 2). (b) Time t_1 is greater than t_2, typical of a spin echo pulse sequence with a short *TE* and a spatial presaturation pulse. Four echoes are formed. Two are used in routine imaging (echoes 1 and 2). The stimulated echo occurs at time $t_1 + t_2$ (echo 3).

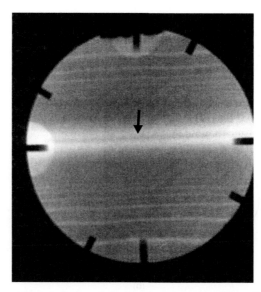

Figure 9.14 Signal contributions from undesired echoes produce banding artifacts (arrow). These echoes can be minimized through the use of coherence spoiling, either gradient-or RF-based.

echoes add in a more incoherent manner. If a sufficiently large number of phase variations is used, the net result is that the undesired signals average to zero. RF spoiling does not require additional time during the slice loop, but does require sophisticated phase modulation of the transmitter (Figure 9.15).

9.2.6 Magnetic susceptibility difference artifact

A third artifact whose appearance is sensitive to the measurement sequence is caused by differences in magnetic susceptibility χ between adjacent regions of tissue. As mentioned in Chapter 1, the magnetic susceptibility is a measure of the spin polarization induced by the external magnetic field. The degree of polarization depends on the electronic and atomic structure of the sample. Tissues such as cortical bone or air-filled organs such as lungs or bowel contain little polarizable material and have very small values for χ. Soft tissue has a greater degree of polarization and larger χ and metallic objects have an even larger χ than soft tissue. At the interface between soft tissues and the area of different susceptibility, a significant change in the local magnetic field is present over a short distance, causing an enhanced dephasing of the protons located there (see Chapter 3). As *TE* increases, there is more time for proton dephasing to occur, which results in signal loss. This dephasing is reversed by the 180° refocusing pulse in spin echo imaging since it is constant with time, but contributes to the contrast in gradient echo imaging (Figure 9.16). Magnetic susceptibility dephasing is also observed following administration of a paramagnetic contrast agent as the agent accumulates in the kidney and bladder. A significant signal loss can occur as the agent concentration in these organs increases (Figure 9.17).

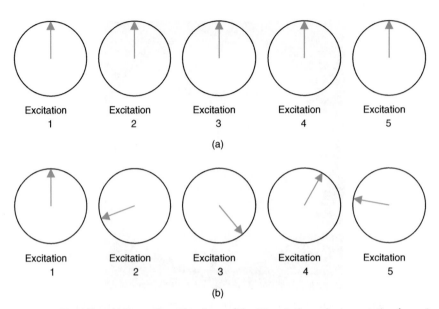

(a)

(b)

Figure 9.15 RF spoiling. (a) No spoiling. The phase of the RF excitation pulse in a rotating frame is the same for all RF pulses. The net magnetization will be rotated along the same axis following each RF excitation pulse. (b) RF spoiling. The phase of the RF excitation pulse in a rotating frame is incremented so that each RF pulse has a different phase. The net magnetization will be rotated along different axes following each RF excitation pulse.

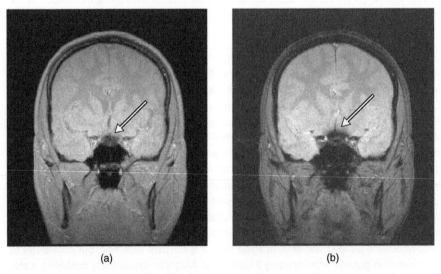

Figure 9.16 Magnetic susceptibility difference artifact. An increase in TE causes increased sensitivity to $T2*$ in gradient echo pulse sequences. Increased distortions occur in areas where there are significant differences in magnetic susceptibility, such as in the posterior fossa (arrows). Other measurement parameters: pulse sequence, two-dimensional spoiled gradient echo; TR, 170 ms; excitation angle, 30°; acquisition matrix, N_{PE}, 224 and N_{RO}, 256; FOV, 201 mm PE × 230 mm RO; N_{SA}, 1. (a) TE, 4 ms; (b) TE, 15 ms.

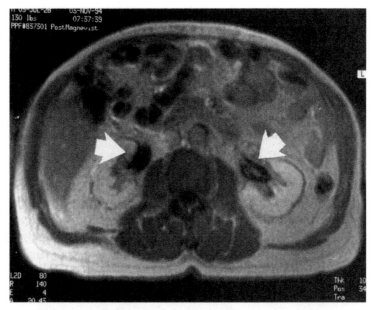

Figure 9.17 Magnetic susceptibility difference artifact. As paramagnetic contrast agents accumulate in the kidneys, the local magnetic field is distorted, causing enhanced dephasing to the protons in the vicinity and produces signal voids (arrows). Measurement parameters are: pulse sequence, two-dimensional spoiled gradient echo; TR, 140 ms; TE, 4 ms; acquisition matrix, N_{PE}, 128 and N_{RO}, 256 with twofold oversampling; FOV, 263 mm PE × 350 mm RO; N_{SA}, 1.

9.2.7 Radial artifact

For radial scanning (see Figure 5.18), an artifact can result if there is an insufficient number of planes sampled. This artifact is sometimes referred to as a "star" or streaking artifact and has a similar artifact found in CT scanning. An inadequate number of planes causes a breakdown in the interpolation process necessary to create the correct k space. The result is a streaking in the reconstructed image (Figure 9.18).

9.3 External artifacts

External artifacts are generated from sources other than patient tissue. Their appearance in the final images depends on the nature of the source and the measurement conditions. The sources may be classified into two general categories: those originating from a malfunctioning or miscalibration of the MRI hardware and those that are not. Excluded from this group are hardware problems that cause complete failure of data collection or image reconstruction. Manufacturers exert great effort to ensure that the acquired images faithfully represent the MR signals from the defined area of interest. The artifacts described here are not specific to any particular manufacturer, but can occur on any MR system.

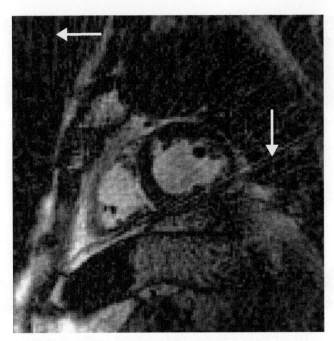

Figure 9.18 Radial artifact. Insufficient number of sample planes in a radial scan produces a scatter or "star" artifact. The primary scatter lines are indicated by the white arrows.

9.3.1 Magnetic field distortions

One of the most common system-related problems is produced by static distortions of the main magnetic field. These distortions may be due to causes related to the magnet environment or to the patient. They can cause contrast variations within the image, particularly when fat saturation is used. External causes may be transient in nature or permanent. Transient causes are typically due to unattached metal inside or near the magnet bore. These may be items such as metal clips or hooks on clothing, or staples or other removable objects. Also, items such as wheelchairs or gurneys may have metal components that alter the magnetic environment and thereby distort the magnet homogeneity. These sources can easily be eliminated by removing the metal from the vicinity of the bore. Permanent distortions to the magnetic field can be caused by metal structures surrounding the magnet (e.g., walls, cabinets) or due to manufacturing imperfections within the magnet itself. During system installation, manufacturers perform a field optimization procedure known as shimming (see Chapter 14) to eliminate coarse distortions of the central magnetic field caused by the permanent structures.

Magnetic field distortions related to the patient are typically of two types. The presence of the patient inside the magnet bore will distort the magnetic field, due to a nonuniform shape and tissue susceptibility. The other source of distortion arises from metal implants. They will deform the local magnetic field homogeneity surrounding the implant, producing significant artifacts. These artifacts frequently appear as an expansive rounded signal void with peripheral areas of high signal intensity distorting the surrounding regions, termed a "blooming" artifact. The size and shape of the artifact depends on the size, shape, orientation, and nature of the metal and the pulse sequence used for the scan (Figure 9.19). Titanium or tantalum

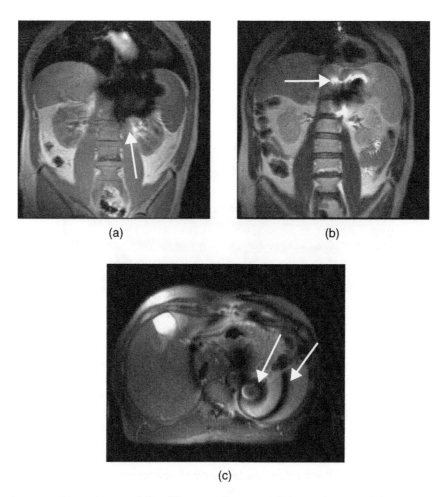

(a)   (b)

(c)

Figure 9.19 Magnetic susceptibility difference artifact. Surgical clips produce a void of signal caused due to the significant magnetic field distortion. (a) Spoiled gradient echo sequence shows significant signal distortion (arrow). (b) Single-shot echo train spin echo at the same level shows less signal loss (arrow). (c) Single-shot echo train spin echo with fat saturation shows incomplete saturation due to field distortions (arrows).

produce very localized distortions, while stainless steel can produce severe distortions that may compromise the images (Figure 9.20). All echoes are affected by the presence of the metal.

The amount of image distortion observed from static field inhomogeneities also depends on the specific measurement technique. If the field homogeneity disruption is severe, the signal loss will be enough to preclude any image whatsoever. In general, gradient echo sequences are most sensitive to field distortions. This is due to the echo signal amplitude being a function of $T2^*$, in which proton dephasing from magnetic field inhomogeneities is a significant factor affecting the image contrast. As in the case of magnetic susceptibility differences discussed earlier, very short TE values allow little time for such dephasing and result in smaller signal voids. Longer TE values allow more time for dephasing and can produce significant artifacts.

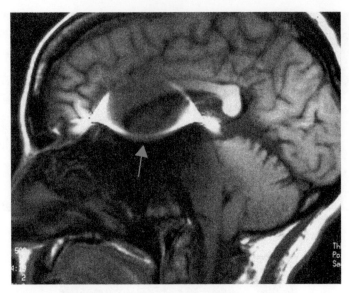

Figure 9.20 Stainless-steel aneurysm clip produces severe field distortion.
Pulse sequence: spin echo.

In some instances, only spin echo sequences may produce acceptable images. Echo train spin echo techniques with short echo spacings are least sensitive to these distortions and should be used when metal is known to be in the imaging field. In addition, common metal objects within the bore, such as clothing clasps, paper clips, or staples, can cause severe image distortion.

Another instance of magnetic field distortion artifacts occurs when fat saturation is used. As mentioned in Chapter 7, fat saturation pulses are RF pulses centered at the fat resonant frequency that saturate the fat protons, leaving only the water protons to contribute to the image. If the field homogeneity is not uniform, the fat resonant frequency may vary within the image. The fat suppression pulse may not uniformly suppress the fat and may even suppress the water within the tissue. This condition results in regions of nonuniform fat suppression within the image (see Figure 8.8b) and is most commonly observed at the edges of the optimized portion of the field, as can occur in images with large FOVs or with extreme superior or inferior positions. It is advisable to try to center the anatomy within the magnet as much as possible and to perform field homogeneity correction (also called "shimming") with the patient inside the scanner prior to fat saturation.

9.3.2 Measurement hardware

Hardware-induced artifacts are those produced by malfunctioning of one or more of the scanner components during the data collection. Most MR techniques acquire multiple signals from the volume of tissue, varying only a single gradient amplitude (the phase encoding gradient) from one measurement to the next. The assumption is that any amplitude variation in the detected signal is caused by the phase encoding gradient, providing the basis for localization in that direction. One of the primary requirements of the measurement hardware for this approach to succeed is that the different subsystems act in a reliable and reproducible fashion. A lack of stability in the performance of any of the system components causes amplitude or phase modulations or distortions in the detected signal in addition to those intrinsic to the measurement. This instability may be electronic in nature, arising from one of the electronic components of the gradient, RF transmitter or receiver, or electrical shim acting in an unreliable or inconsistent manner. It may also be mechanical in nature if the magnet, patient table, or receiver coil are not supported properly. In this case, the pulsing of the gradient coil causes motion of the patient relative to the receiver coil. The signal distortions result in smearing or ghosting artifacts in the phase encoding direction throughout the entire image field. The magnitude and nature of the instability determines the amount of smearing. In many instances, the instability artifacts are indistinguishable from motion artifacts. Manufacturers perform tests during system calibration to assess the stability of the various systems to ensure that their performance is reproducible and stable.

Proper calibration of the measurement hardware is another important contribution to high-quality MR imaging. The gradient, RF transmitter, and receiver systems are calibrated to ensure their proper performance. Improper calibration produces variable distortions, depending on which component is considered. Nonlinear gradient pulses or incorrect amplitude calibration cause incorrect spatial localization and/or image distortion. Improper RF calibration causes incorrect or nonuniform excitation power, which may or may not be noticeable in the

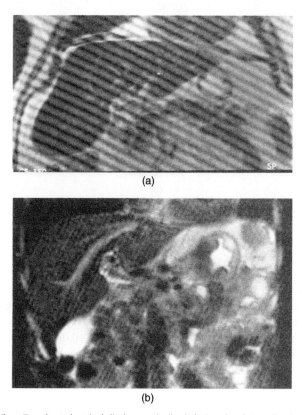

(a)

(b)

Figure 9.21 Spikes. Transient electrical discharges (spikes) during the data collection period produce a banding pattern that is superimposed across the entire imaging field. The direction and spacing of the bands depend on the timing of the discharge relative to the collection of the central phase-encoding steps.

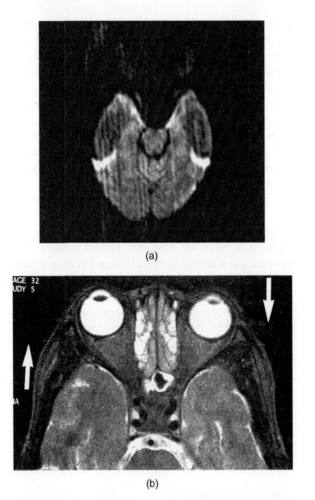

(a)

(b)

Figure 9.22 External interference: (a) artifact due to electrical source outside the scan room; (b) interference from portable patient medication unit operating in scan room during the measurement (arrows).

resulting images. The RF power deposition as measured by the specific absorption rate (SAR) will also be inaccurate. Receiver miscalibration causes incorrect amplification of the echo signal, which may result in insufficient gain so that the signal does not exceed the background noise or in excessive gain, which may cause the echo signal to exceed the digitization limits of the scanner. If parallel acquisition techniques are used, then improper balancing of the individual receiver channels can cause intensity distortions. Verification of system calibrations is normally performed during preventive maintenance of the scanner.

9.3.3 Noise

A final artifact often present in MR images is noise. Noise can have a variety of appearances, depending on the origin and nature of the source. It may appear as a film superimposed over the normal anatomy, with or without discernible patterns, or it may have a discrete pattern or patterns. The two most common examples of coherent noise are spikes and those arising from external sources.

Spikes are noise bursts of short duration that occur randomly during the data collection. They are normally caused by static electricity discharges or arcing of electrical components, but may be generated by many different sources. Their appearance in an image depends on the severity, number, and location of the spike in relation to the signal maximum, but tend to appear as waves superimposed on the normal image data, including waves in the background (Figure 9.21). They may or may not occur in all images of the scan. Spikes are particularly problematic to isolate because they are often irreproducible, particularly if the source is static discharge.

External interference artifacts occur when there is a source of time-varying signal detected by the receiver. They appear as lines of constant frequency within the image. Their positions depend on the receiver bandwidth of the sequence and the frequency difference from the transmitter. The most common example of this is from the alternating nature (AC) of standard electrical current (60 Hz in the United States, 50 Hz in Europe and Asia) (Figure 9.22). Electrical connections for any equipment, such as external patient monitoring devices used in the scanner room, should be filtered before being allowed to penetrate the Faraday shield or the use of nonalternating (DC) current should be considered. Manufacturers should be consulted before incorporating any electrical equipment into the scan room to ensure compatibility with the MR scanner.

CHAPTER 10

Motion artifact reduction techniques

As discussed in Chapter 9, motion in an MR image can produce severe image artifacts in the phase encoding direction. The severity of the artifact depends on the nature of the motion, the time during data collection when the motion occurs, and the particular pulse sequence and measurement parameters. The most critical portion of the data collection period for artifact generation is during the measurement of echoes following low-amplitude phase encoding steps (center of k-space). Motion during the high-amplitude phase encoding steps (edges of k-space) can cause blurring but not severe signal misregistration in the image.

Four methods are commonly used to reduce the severity of the motion artifact on the final image. If signal from the moving tissue is not of interest, use of a spatial presaturation pulse as described in Chapter 8 can significantly reduce artifactual signal. This is useful to suppress abdominal or cardiac motion artifacts in spine examinations. The other techniques are useful when signal from the moving tissue is desired. Two of these, acquisition parameter modification and physiological triggering, affect the mechanics of the data collection process, while the third method, flow compensation, alters the intrinsic signal from the moving tissue. Although none of these approaches completely removes motion artifacts from the image, use of one or more of these techniques substantially reduces the impact of motion on the final images.

10.1 Acquisition parameter modification

Proper choice of the acquisition parameters can alter the appearance of motion artifacts. One example of this is to define the phase encoding direction so that the motion artifact does not obscure the area of interest. This may be referred to as motion artifact rotation or swapping the frequency and phase encoding directions as the physical gradient directions for PE and RO are switched. This approach does not eliminate or minimize the artifact, but only changes its position within the image. For example, motion artifacts due to eye movement or blood flow from the sagittal sinus vein may obscure lesions in the cerebrum if

---

MRI Basic Principles and Applications, Fifth Edition.
Brian M. Dale, Mark A. Brown and Richard C. Semelka.
© 2015 John Wiley & Sons, Ltd. Published 2015 by John Wiley & Sons, Ltd.

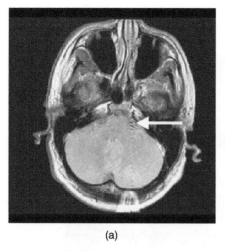 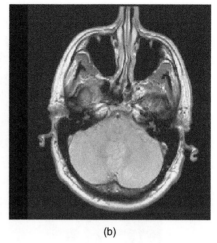

(a)   (b)

Figure 10.1 The direction of motion artifacts is determined by the phase-encoding gradient. Blood flow during the scan produces motion artifact (arrow). (a) RO: left/right, PE: anterior/posterior; (b) RO: anterior/posterior, PE: left/right.

the phase encoding direction for a transverse slice is in the anterior–posterior direction. If the phase encoding direction is in the left–right direction, the eye motion artifacts lie outside the brain. The blood flow artifact also appears in an area outside the brain (Figure 10.1).

Another example of parameter modification is to increase the number of signal averages. This approach is of particular benefit in abdominal imaging where respiratory motion can produce severe ghosting. With multiple averages, the signal from the tissue is based on its average position throughout the scan. Since the tissue is in the same location most of the time, the signals add coherently. The motion artifact signal will be reduced in amplitude relative to the tissue signal.

Alternately, removal of respiratory artifacts in abdominal or cardiac imaging can be accomplished by measuring all the scan data within one breath-hold. For example, a $TR = 140$ ms, $N_{PE} = 128$, and $N_{SA} = 1$ can produce a complete scan in 18 seconds. The spatial resolution may be compromised in the phase encoding direction, depending on the FOV_{PE}, but respiratory motion and its artifacts will not be present if the patient suspends respiration. Extreme examples of this approach are single-shot echo train spin echo and EPI techniques, where images can be acquired in less than one second, producing heart and bowel images that are virtually motion–artifact free (Figure 10.2).

10.2 Triggering/Gating

Another method for visualizing moving tissue allows the tissue to move but synchronizes the data collection with a periodic signal produced by the patient, such

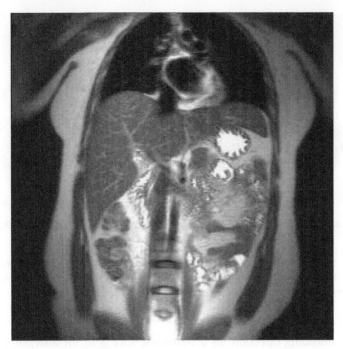

Figure 10.2 Single-shot echo train spin echo image of abdomen. Note lack of motion artifact from heart and bowel.

as a pulse or heartbeat. The data collection–timing signal relationship can be exploited in two ways. Prospective methods initiate the data collection following detection of the timing signal. The signal detection for a particular slice always occurs at the same time following the timing signal. Since the moving tissue is in the same relative position at this time, there is minimal misregistration of the signal and a significant reduction of the resulting motion artifact. Retrospective methods measure the timing signal together with the echo signal, but the timing signal is not analyzed nor the measured data adjusted until the scan is completed. The data collection process can also be triggered by or gated to the timing signal.

Triggering examinations are commonly prospective in nature and begin the data collection following detection of a signal. The noise produced by the scanner during sequence execution is also synchronized to the signal source. The *TR* controlling the contrast is based on the repetition time for the trigger signal T_{REP} rather than the *TR* entered in the user interface. Several external methods for detection of the timing signal can be used. For cardiac imaging, data collection is synchronized to the electrocardiogram (ECG) signal measured from the patient using lead wires. Pulse triggering uses a pulse sensor to detect the pulse, usually measured on an extremity. Respiratory triggering uses a pressure or strain transducer attached to the patient to measure either chest or abdominal motion. An internal method for a timing reference uses a so-called "navigator echo" that, when properly positioned, can measure an MR signal from the diaphragm or other tissue and indicate that motion has occurred.

There are several potential problems with triggered studies. One is that the scan time is longer for a triggered study than for the corresponding untriggered study. Time must be allowed from the end of data collection (traditionally TR) to the next trigger signal to ensure that the trigger signal is properly detected by the measurement hardware. This extra time is usually 150–200 ms to allow for variation of the rate of the trigger signal for the patient. The total scan time will be extended by approximately 1–2 minutes. Another problem occurs if the rate of the trigger signal is irregular. The T_{REP} for a particular phase encoding step depends on the R–R time interval immediately prior to the step under consideration. Variation in the heart rate causes variation in the amount of $T1$ relaxation from measurement to measurement for each phase encoding step. This variation produces amplitude changes in the detected signal, producing misregistration artifacts in the final images even if the triggering is perfect. Stability of the heart rate is most critical during collection of the echoes around the k-space center ($k_y = 0$).

Cardiac examinations are one example of an examination that typically uses prospective triggering. The peak R wave is normally used as the timing reference point. Each phase encoding step is acquired at the same point in time following the R wave so that the heart is in the same relative position (Figure 10.3). Since the kernel time per slice is shorter than the duration of the R–R interval (T_{REP}), several signals can be acquired within one heartbeat. Proper detection of the ECG signal from the patient is critical. Improper electrode placement may detect significant signal from the blood during its flow through the aortic arch. In addition, the transmitted RF energy and the gradient pulses may also interact with the lead wires, inducing significant noise to the detected ECG signal. High-resistance lead wires may even burn the patient through this coupling.

Historically, triggered examinations used spin echo sequences for data collection, in which one signal (line of k-space) was acquired per slice per heartbeat. Each image within the scan is acquired at a different position and a different time point in the cardiac cycle. These images were typically $T1$-weighted (depending on the R–R time interval) with a minimal blood signal and were used for morphological studies of the heart. Current scan techniques use gradient echo sequences in a segmented manner to acquire multiple lines of k-space per slice per heartbeat. This allows a complete raw data set to be acquired in fewer heartbeats, which reduces the scan sensitivity to a variable heart rate. In many cases, the scan times are short enough for patients to suspend respiration, which reduces artifacts from respiratory motion. These scans may use a spoiled gradient echo sequence to produce morphologic images (Figure 10.4), or a partially or totally refocused gradient echo sequence to produce images with a bright blood signal. Rapid display of these images allows a dynamic or cine visualization of the heart and cardiac hemodynamics during the different phases of the cardiac

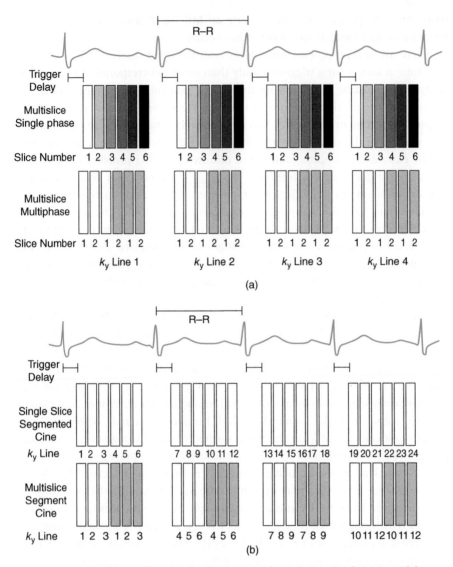

Figure 10.3 Triggered data collection. The R wave is used as a timing signal. A trigger delay (TD) can be used to initiate data collection at any time desired during the cardiac cycle. (a) Nonsegmented measurement. For multislice single-phase imaging, one k_y line for each slice is acquired per heartbeat. Information for a particular slice is acquired at the same time following the R wave. The *T1* contrast is based on the R–R time interval rather than the user-defined *TR*. Alternatively, a multislice, multiphase acquisition may be carried out in which slices are acquired at different times during the cardiac cycle at the same position. (b) Segmented measurement. For single-slice imaging, multiple k_y lines are acquired for a particular slice following the R wave. For multislice imaging, multiple k_y lines are acquired for multiple slices following the R wave.

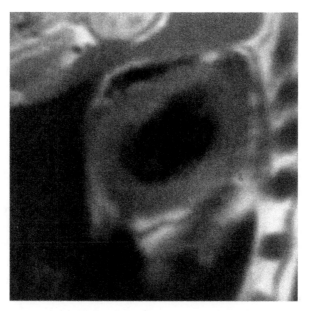

Figure 10.4 Short-axis $T1$-weighted image acquired using a triggered multislice mode.

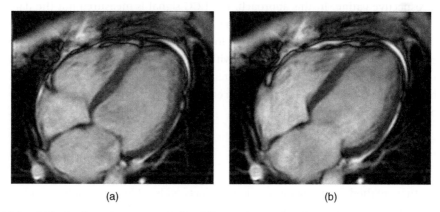

(a)   (b)

Figure 10.5 Cine heart images acquired at different phases of cardiac cycle. Measurement parameters: pulse sequence, two-dimensional spoiled gradient echo; TR, 35.4 ms; TE, 1.5 ms; excitation angle, 65°; acquisition matrix, N_{PE}, 108 and N_{RO}, 128; FOV, 169 mm PE × 200 mm RO; N_{SA}, 1. (a) 92 ms following R wave; (b) 552 ms following R wave.

cycle (Figure 10.5). Prospective cine examinations have a problem that the initial image in the data set, representing the first phase of the cardiac cycle for the scan, will often be brighter than the subsequent images in the scan. This is due to the longer amount of $T1$ relaxation that the net magnetization undergoes for this time point compared to the other images, due to the "dead" time waiting for the trigger pulse.

Gating methods typically have the sequence continuously executing RF and gradient pulses but not measuring signal, and link the timing signal to the time when echoes are actually measured. The continuous execution maintains a relatively constant net magnetization so that all images will have comparable contrast. Prospective gating has been used in cardiac imaging and in abdominal imaging to reduce artifacts from respiratory motion. Two approaches are used, both of which synchronize the data collection to the respiratory cycle of the patient. Simple respiratory gating acquires the data when there is minimal motion. It suffers from significantly longer scan times since the time during respiratory motion is not used for data collection. An alternative technique used for $T1$-weighted imaging, respiratory compensation, rearranges the order of phase encoding so that adjacent G_{PE} are acquired when the abdomen is in the same relative position. Typically, the low-amplitude G_{PE} are acquired at or near end expiration so that the echoes contributing the most signals are measured when there is the least motion. Higher amplitude G_{PE} are acquired during inspiration. Significant improvement of respiratory-induced ghosts can be achieved by either technique as long as there is a uniform respiration rate during the scan. Nonuniform respiration may produce artifacts as severe as those produced from a nongated scan.

An alternative to prospective triggering for cine heart imaging is known as retrospective gating. In this approach, the ECG signal is measured but the data collection is not controlled by the timing signal. Instead, the data are measured in an untriggered fashion and the time following the R wave when each phase encoding step was measured is stored with it. Following completion of the data collection, images are reconstructed corresponding to various time points within the cardiac cycle. The data for any phase encoding step not directly measured are interpolated from the measured values.

10.3 Flow compensation

Another method for reducing motion artifacts adds additional gradient pulses to the pulse sequence to correct for phase shifts experienced by the moving protons. It is known as flow compensation, gradient motion rephasing (GMR), or the motion artifact suppression technique (MAST). As described in Chapter 6, gradient pulses of equal area but opposite polarity are used to generate a gradient echo. Proper dephasing and rephasing of the protons and correct frequency and phase mapping occur as long as there is no motion during the gradient pulses. Movement during either gradient pulse results in incomplete phase cancellation or a net phase accumulation at the end of the second gradient pulse time. The amount of phase accumulation is a function of the velocity of the motion. This residual phase accumulation produces signal intensity variations that are manifest as motion artifacts in the phase encoding direction (Figure 10.6a), regardless of the direction of the motion or the gradient pulses.

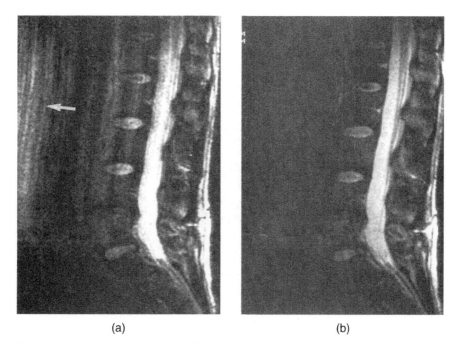

(a)   (b)

Figure 10.6 Flow compensation. Use of flow compensation gradient pulses will map moving protons such as cerebrospinal fluid to their proper location. Measurement parameters are: pulse sequence, spin echo; TR, 2500 ms; TE, 90 ms; excitation angle, 90°; acquisition matrix, N_{PE}, 192 and N_{RO}, 256 with twofold readout oversampling; FOV, 210 mm PE × 280 mm RO; N_{SA}, 1; slice thickness, 5 mm. (a) No flow compensation. Misregistration artifact from CSF flow appears anterior to the spinal canal (arrow). (b) First-order flow compensation in readout and slice-selection directions. CSF is properly mapped into the spinal canal.

If the velocity of the protons is approximately constant during the gradient pulse then the motion-induced phase changes can be corrected by applying additional gradient pulses. These pulses will be applied in the direction for which compensation is desired. The duration, amplitude, and timing of the pulses can be defined so that protons moving with constant velocity can be properly mapped within the image, and similar methods exist for acceleration, etc. (Pipe and Chenevert, 1991). For gradient echo sequences, velocity compensation is normally sufficient for proper registration of cerebrospinal fluid, while for spin echo sequences, higher order compensation can often be achieved with minimal complications (Figure 10.6b).

Flow compensation requires that certain limitations be placed on the pulse sequence. Since additional gradient pulses are applied during the slice loop, the minimum TE for the sequence must be extended to allow time for their application. In pulse sequences where short TEs are desired, higher amplitude gradient pulses of shorter duration may be used. This will limit the minimum FOV available for the sequence. In practice, only modest increases in TE and the minimum FOV are normally required.

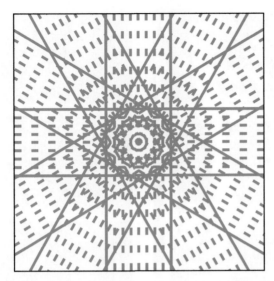

Figure 10.7 Radial motion compensation. Each scan measures a portion of k-space (dark lines). Some of the measured lines contain points acquired at the center of k-space.

10.4 Radial-based motion compensation

A final method for motion compensation is based on the fact that radial scanning always acquires data through the center of k-space. These lines can be used to correct for in-plane motion in the image, as the points near the center should have a comparable signal regardless of the gradient direction. One method of data collection uses a segmented data collection as in echo train spin echo, except that each echo train acquires lines of data near the center of k-space at different angles (view directions) (Figure 10.7). This method, known as PROPELLER or BLADE, creates an image of low spatial resolution to correct for motion. It requires a regridding of the data to ensure that there are no gaps in the raw data, but can produce images with good image quality with minimal motion artifact.

CHAPTER 11

Magnetic resonance angiography

One of the strengths of MRI for imaging patient tissue is its ability to acquire information regarding its function as well as its structure. The most common example is the examination of flowing blood within the vascular network using MR angiography (MRA). In Chapter 9, moving tissue was shown to produce severe image artifacts. MRA uses flowing tissue such as blood to provide the primary source of signal intensity in the image. It allows visualization of the normal, laminar flow of blood within the vascular system and its disruptions due to pathologic conditions such as stenoses or occlusions. MRA can be of particular benefit in evaluating vessel patency. MRA techniques have the advantage over conventional X-ray-based angiographic techniques in that use of a contrast agent is not always required. Consequently, multiple scans may be performed if desired (e.g., visualizing arterial and then venous flow).

The most common MRA approach is known as a "bright-blood" technique. A signal from the moving protons is accentuated relative to the stationary protons through the pulse sequence and measurement parameters. Whether the vessels are displayed as white pixels on a dark background or dark pixels on a bright background, bright-blood MRA techniques assign high pixel amplitudes to the laminar-flowing blood. Bright-blood MRA techniques can be divided into two approaches: time-of-flight and phase contrast methods. In their simplest implementation, both methods visualize arterial and venous flow simultaneously through the volume of interest. This can lead to an ambiguous identification if the vessels are in close proximity to each other. One approach to select either arterial or venous flow is to apply spatial presaturation pulses to saturate the undesired blood signal prior to its entry into the imaging volume (Figure 11.1). Presaturation pulses may also be used in "black blood" MRA techniques where the blood signal is saturated and the vessels appear dark relative to the surrounding tissue. These techniques are seldom used and will not be discussed further in this book.

MRA techniques use gradient echo sequences as the measurement technique for data collection and may use 2D sequential slice (number of slices equal to the number of subloops) or 3D volume acquisition modes. Gradient echo sequences

MRI Basic Principles and Applications, Fifth Edition.
Brian M. Dale, Mark A. Brown and Richard C. Semelka.
© 2015 John Wiley & Sons, Ltd. Published 2015 by John Wiley & Sons, Ltd.

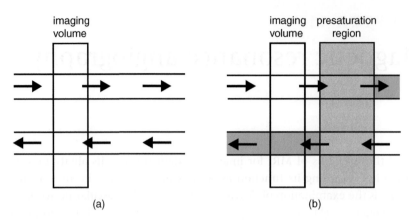

Figure 11.1 Flow selection in MR angiography. (a) In the absence of a spatial presaturation pulse, flowing blood entering the imaging volume is visualized regardless of the direction of the flow. (b) A spatial presaturation pulse that saturates flowing blood prior to its entry into the imaging volume suppresses signal from that volume.

allow the use of short *TE* times (usually less than 10 ms), which minimize *T2** dephasing of the blood and other tissues. The choice of a 2D versus a 3D technique is usually dictated based on the total volume of tissue to be examined and by the total scan time. Three-dimensional techniques provide the best spatial resolution in all three directions and minimize vessel misregistration artifacts. However, saturation of blood at the distal side of the excitation volume limits the volume to approximately 70 mm unless a *T1* relaxation agent is used. The improved spatial resolution of 3D methods requires significantly longer scan times. The 2D method is preferable for imaging vessels with slow flow velocity, such as veins, or to limit saturation effects from the in-plane flow. Coverage of large areas of anatomy is possible in one scan since the volume of excitation is typically 3–4 mm per slice.

There are two additional problems associated with MRA. One is that the saturation pulse becomes less effective as more time elapses between the presaturation and the excitation pulses. This problem occurs both due to increased *T1* relaxation of the blood as well as time-of-flight effects (see Section 11.1). This loss of effectiveness can be minimized by proper positioning of the saturation pulse near the volume of excitation. Care must be taken in positioning if there is pulsatile flow in the vessel of interest, as too close a position to the imaging volume could cause a reduction in the signal if the flow is retrograde in nature. A second problem is an exaggerated sensitivity to vessel stenosis. The stenotic region disrupts the laminar flow in the area of and distal to the stenosis, causing a loss of vessel signal to a greater extent than from the stenotic region alone. As the laminar flow is reestablished within the vessel, a bright signal can again be measured, demonstrating patency of the vessel.

11.1 Time-of-flight MRA

Time-of-flight techniques are the most time-efficient methods for obtaining MRA images. A single measurement is performed, with the stationary tissue signal suppressed relative to the flowing tissue signal for the imaging volume. A moderate excitation pulse angle and a *TR* much shorter than the tissue *T1* values are used to accomplish this. While the stationary tissue experiences every RF excitation pulse, the flowing tissue does not. A volume of blood will be at a different location at the time of each excitation pulse due to its motion during *TR* (Figure 11.2). The signal from the blood volume is largest at the entry point of the slice because it has not undergone any excitation pulses. As the blood volume travels through the slice, it becomes progressively saturated as it undergoes more excitation pulses and loses signal. If the flow direction is perpendicular to the slice (through-plane flow) and the volume of excitation is small, then the volume of blood exits the slice before it is completely saturated and a significant blood signal can be measured throughout the entire slice. If the flow is contained within the excitation volume (in-plane flow), then significant saturation of the blood will occur and the blood signal will be isointense with the stationary tissue unless a *T1* relaxation agent is used. The degree of blood saturation depends on the slice thickness, *TR*, excitation angle, and flow velocity.

Time-of-flight techniques suffer from two limitations. One is that it provides only a qualitative assessment of flow velocity. The second problem is that

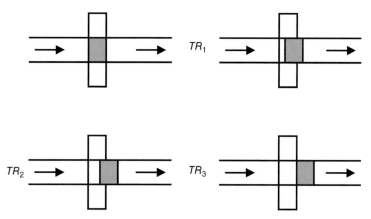

Figure 11.2 Time-of-flight effect. During data collection, the imaging volume experiences multiple RF pulses. Flowing blood (colored box) experiences the first RF pulse (upper left). During the first *TR* period, the excited blood volume moves (upper right) and only a portion experiences the second RF pulse. During the second *TR* time period, the initial volume of blood continues to move (lower left). By the end of a third *TR* time period, the initial volume of blood is entirely outside the volume of excitation and does not contribute to the detected signal (lower right).

there is incomplete suppression of the background tissue due to the faster $T1$ relaxation times of the stationary tissues relative to the blood, particularly fat. Magnetization transfer (MT) pulses are often incorporated for additional suppression of the stationary tissue water to enhance the ability for small vessel detection at the expense of increased TR and relative fat signal (Figure 11.3). Three-dimensional time-of-flight techniques produce increased saturation of the blood due to the large number of excitation pulses of the imaging volume. For this reason, they are suitable only for visualizing vessels with fast flow velocities, such as moderate-sized arteries.

Two approaches have been developed to overcome this saturation. For 3D examinations with through-plane flow, the excitation pulse can be modified to produce a ramped or nonuniform range of excitation angles across the imaging volume (Figure 11.4). The effective excitation ramp is oriented so that increased energy is applied to protons located at the distal side of the imaging volume. This induces more transverse magnetization and more signal from the more saturated protons (Figure 11.5). A second approach is analogous to traditional X-ray angiography and is used for examinations with in-plane flow such as the visualization of pulmonary or abdominal arteries. $T1$ contrast agents can be administered as a bolus to shorten the $T1$ relaxation time of blood and obtain more blood signal (Figure 11.6). Measurement times can be reduced to a few seconds through the use of interpolation in the slice selection. These short times will enable serial scan volumes coupled with suspension of respiration to be acquired during the measurement. Subtraction of pre- and postcontrast volumes eliminates the residual signal from stationary tissue. Use of contrast agents for abdominal MRA has enabled rapid, reliable, and high-quality studies to be obtained with minimal contamination from patient motion. Studies of peripheral vessels by MRA can also be performed following contrast administration (Figure 11.7). However, caution must be used in the use of contrast media in patients with compromised renal function (see Chapter 15).

While the use of contrast media aids in MRA examinations of anatomy that can be acquired in a single-scan volume, its use for scanning larger anatomical regions such as peripheral vessels in the lower extremities or for dynamic examinations is problematic. The timing when contrast media is in the anatomical area of interest can be short for arterial vessels. To achieve images with good spatial resolution as well as good temporal resolution, techniques have been developed that do not scan k-space uniformly in time; in other words, those lines of k-space that primarily determine contrast (low amplitude k_y/k_z) are acquired more frequently than those that primarily affect spatial resolution (high amplitude k_y/k_z). The signals from the high amplitude k_y/k_z lines are used in multiple data sets to create images with less inter-set time variation. These techniques are known as TWIST (Time-Resolved Angiography with Interleaved Stochastic Trajectories), TRICKS (Time-Resolved Imaging of Contrast Kinetics), or 4D-TRAK (4D Time-Resolved MR Angiography with Keyhole).

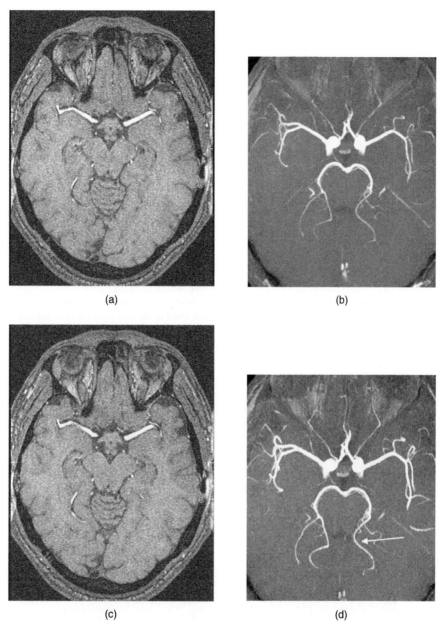

(a)

(b)

(c)

(d)

Figure 11.3 Time-of-flight MRA showing effects of magnetization transfer pulse. Other measurement parameters are: pulse sequence, three-dimensional refocused gradient echo, post excitation; *TR*, 42 ms; *TE*, 7 ms; excitation angle, 25°; acquisition matrix, N_{PE}, 192 and N_{RO}, 512 with twofold readout oversampling; FOV, 201 mm PE × 230 mm RO; N_{SA}, 1; effective slice thickness, 0.78 mm. (a) Source image, one from data set acquired without MT pulse; (b) transverse post processed image of (a); (c) source image, one from data set acquired with MT pulse; (d) transverse post processed image of (c). Note reduction of background gray and white matter in (c) compared to (a) and improved visualization of vessels in (d) compared to (b) (arrow).

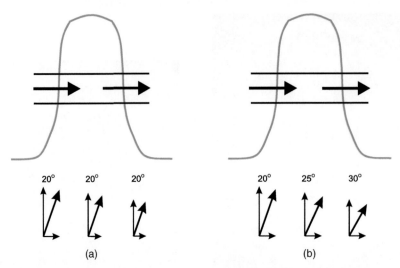

Figure 11.4 TONE RF pulse. (a) Standard excitation pulses provide uniform energy deposition across the slice, which gradually increases saturation of, and reduces the transverse magnetization from, blood located at the exit side of the slice, causing a loss of signal. (b) Nonuniform excitation pulses known as ramped or tilted optimized nonuniform excitation (TONE) RF pulses increase the excitation across the slice. Although the amount of saturation increases, the resulting transverse magnetization remains constant, so that the blood signal remains uniform throughout the imaging volume.

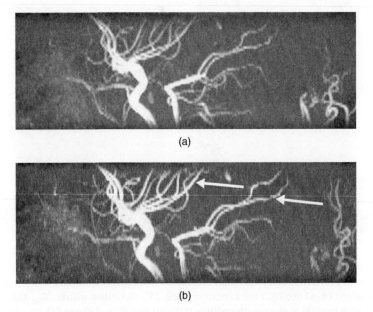

Figure 11.5 Time-of-flight MRA showing effects of TONE RF pulse. Measurement parameters are: pulse sequence, three-dimensional refocused gradient echo, post excitation; TR, 42 ms; TE, 7 ms; excitation angle, 25°; acquisition matrix, N_{PE}, 192 and N_{RO}, 512 with twofold readout oversampling; FOV, 201 mm PE × 230 mm RO; N_{SA}, 1; effective slice thickness, 0.78 mm. (a) Sagittal projection of volume using normal uniform excitation pulse; (b) sagittal projection of volume using TONE excitation pulse. Note improved signal from vessels (arrow).

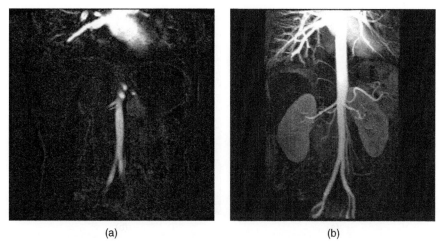

(a)   (b)

Figure 11.6 MR angiography of aorta and renal arteries following bolus administration of gadolinium–chelate contrast agent. Measurement parameters are: pulse sequence, three-dimensional refocused gradient echo, postexcitation; TR, 3 ms; TE, 1.1 ms; excitation angle, 20°; acquisition matrix, N_{PE}, 128 and N_{RO}, 256; FOV, 350 mm PE × 400 mm RO; N_{SA}, 1; effective slice thickness, 2.0 mm. (a) Source image, one from data set. Image was obtained following subtraction of unenhanced scan from enhanced scan. (b) Coronal maximum intensity projection image of (a).

11.2 Phase contrast MRA

Phase contrast MRA is a technique in which the background tissue signal is subtracted from a flow-enhanced image to produce flow-only images. The acquisition sequence may produce a one-dimensional profile, or standard 2D or 3D images. A minimum of two images is measured at each slice position. One image, known as the reference image, is acquired with flow compensation (see Chapter 10). Subsequent images are acquired following application of additional gradient pulses that induce a phase shift in blood moving with a particular direction and flow velocity. The moving protons in the chosen direction are rephased at the echo time TE and the resultant complex or phase image is subtracted from the reference complex or phase image to produce images of only the moving protons. In the complex difference image, the signal amplitude of the blood will depend on its velocity, with a maximum signal obtained from flowing blood with an operator-specified velocity known as the velocity encoding value (V_{enc}). In the phase difference image the pixel values will be proportional to the blood velocity, within a maximum range determined by the V_{enc}. Additional scans may be performed to sensitize flow in other directions or at other velocities. The resultant difference images may be combined to produce images sensitive to flow in any direction (Figure 11.8).

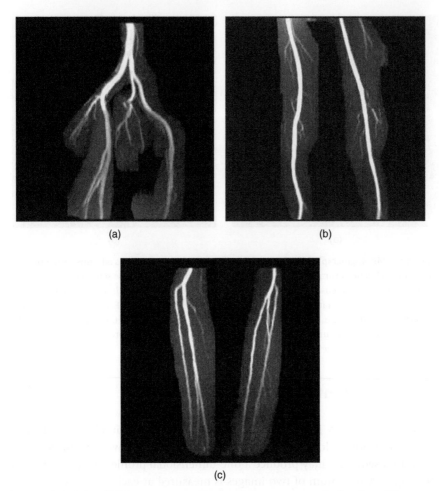

(a) (b)

(c)

Figure 11.7 Peripheral MRA, postprocessed images. Images were acquired at three different scan table positions. Measurement parameters: pulse sequence, two-dimensional spoiled gradient echo; TR, 300 ms: TE, 3.6 ms; excitation angle, 50°; acquisition matrix, N_{PE}, 144 and N_{RO}, 256; FOV, 191 mm PE × 340 mm RO; N_{SA}, 1; slice thickness, 4.0 mm; pulse triggered. (Reproduced with permission of H. Cecil Charles, Duke University.)

Phase contrast MRA has several advantages over time-of-flight techniques. Being subtraction rather than saturation techniques, they have better background suppression than time-of-flight methods. Through their directional sensitization, phase contrast methods also enable flow in each primary direction to be separately assessed. Finally, quantitation of the flow velocity in each direction is possible. However, phase contrast methods suffer from two problems. One is a significantly longer scan time. Four separate acquisitions are required to measure flow in all three directions. The scan time is four times longer than for a time-of-flight method with similar acquisition parameters. In addition, prior knowledge of the maximum velocity is necessary to ensure that the proper

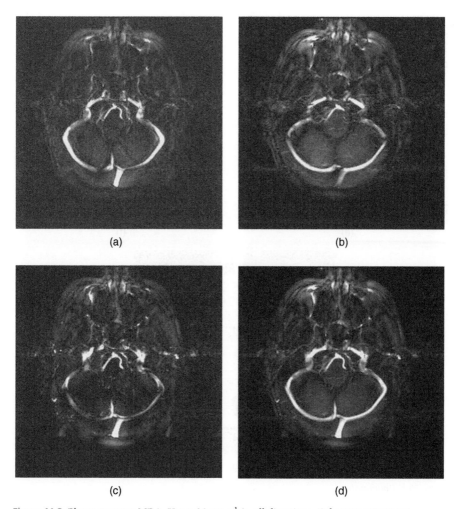

(a)   (b)

(c)   (d)

Figure 11.8 Phase-contrast MRA. Venc, $30\,\mathrm{cm\,s^{-1}}$ in all directions. Other measurement parameters: pulse sequence, two-dimensional spoiled gradient echo; *TR*, 211 ms; *TE*, 8.4 ms; excitation angle, 15°; acquisition matrix, N_{PE}, 192 and N_{RO}, 256; FOV, 240 mm PE × 240 mm RO; N_{SA}, 1; slice thickness, 40.0 mm. (a) Flow image, flow direction A–P; (b) flow image, flow direction R–L; (c) flow image, flow direction S–I; (d) magnitude sum of images (a) to (c); (e) phase image, flow direction A–P; (f) phase image, flow direction R–L; (g) phase image, flow direction S–I.

V_{enc} is used. The maximum signal in the complex difference image is achieved for blood flowing at the chosen V_{enc}. Flow velocities exceeding this velocity are misregistered in the image and appear as slower flow, a situation known as flow aliasing (for instance, a V_{enc} of $30\,\mathrm{cm\,s^{-1}}$ will have equal signal amplitudes for blood flowing at 25 and $35\,\mathrm{cm\,s^{-1}}$). Flow aliasing is analogous to the high-frequency aliasing problem observed in phase encoding (see Chapter 5). The blood signal is reduced at these higher velocities until a complete loss of the

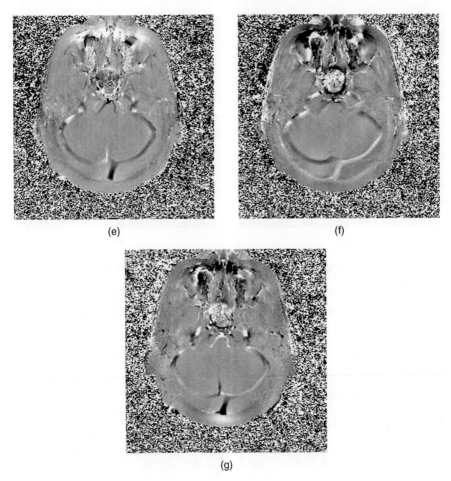

(e)   (f)

(g)

Figure 11.8 (*continued*)

flow signal occurs at flow velocities that are even multiples of the V_{enc}. At the other extreme, a V_{enc} too large will minimize contrast between velocity changes within a vessel (for example, at 30 or 35 cm s^{-1} flow for a V_{enc} of 90 cm s^{-1}). Proper choice of the V_{enc} allows adequate visualization of all flow with good sensitivity to velocity variations within a vessel. This choice can be facilitated by the use of velocity measurements measured using Doppler ultrasound techniques or by scanning the volume using 2D techniques with multiple V_{enc} values to see which one provides the best results.

11.3 Maximum intensity projection

Regardless of the choice of acquisition method, examination of the individual images from an MRA scan is recommended as they can provide details regarding flow variations within a vessel. However, a vessel is seldom located within a single slice but usually extends through several slices at an arbitrary angle, making the vessel tortuosity and the spatial relationship between vessels difficult to assess, particularly if the vessels are oriented perpendicular to the imaging volume. Bright-blood MRA images may be analyzed using a postprocessing technique known as maximum intensity projection (MIP) to better visualize the three-dimensional vessel topography.

The MIP process generates images frequently from the entire set of MRA images. A view direction is chosen and the entire set of images is projected along that direction on to a perpendicular plane using a "ray tracing" approach. The pixel of maximum intensity along the ray is chosen as the pixel for the MIP image, regardless of the input slice where the pixel is located (Figure 11.9). Because the bright-blood MRA technique accentuates the blood signal over the stationary tissue signal, the MIP process preferentially selects blood vessels whenever encountered, enabling the entire vessel to be examined no matter where it is located within the imaging volume. Multiple images may be obtained from the same data set through a change of the view direction (rotation of the projection angle). Vessels that are superimposed in one projection may be clearly resolved in another one. It is also possible to perform the MIP process on a subset of the data, a so-called "targeted" approach. This method is useful for isolating the left and right carotid arteries, for elimination of suborbital or subcutaneous fat in cerebral MRA studies, or for tailored reconstruction of the renal arteries. Care must

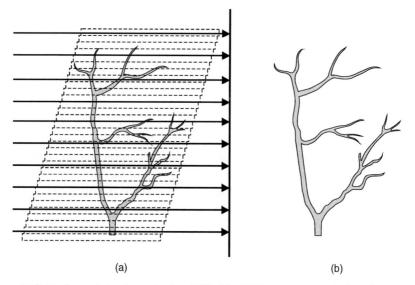

(a)   (b)

Figure 11.9 Maximum intensity projection (MIP). The MR images are acquired so that moving blood has pixels of maximal intensity. The MIP process maps the pixels of maximum intensity into a single projection or view, regardless of which slice the pixel was located in. Changing the direction of projection provides a different perspective of the vessels.

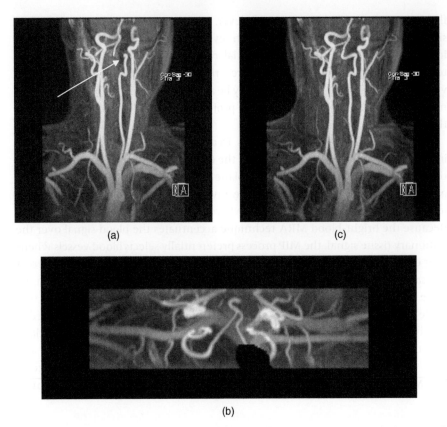

Figure 11.10 Maximum intensity projection. Note lack of vessel in (a) (arrow), which is caused by improper exclusion (b). Processing of the complete data set shows the entire vessel (c).

be taken in the definition of the targeted area that the vessel of interest does not leave the area. The MIP process causes the vessel to be cut off at the edge of the defined region, simulating a vessel occlusion (Figure 11.10). Careful examination of the source images and/or MIP images in multiple orientations is necessary to ensure the inclusion of the entire vessel within the reconstructed area.

Another post-processing approach is known as segmentation. It uses an operator-selected region known as a "seed" region to identify the vessel. The seed region is expanded to include high-intensity pixels in contiguous regions. Since the MRA scan techniques accentuates the blood signal, the vessels will be preferentially chosen. This approach depends on adequate contrast between the blood and the tissue near the vessel.

CHAPTER 12

Advanced imaging applications

Initially, MR imaging was restricted to visualizing hydrogen nuclei using basic spin echo techniques. As hardware and software have evolved, newer and faster imaging techniques have been developed. The advent of subsecond imaging techniques has provided the ability to measure metabolic processes within tissues with significantly faster temporal resolution than was previously possible. Also, imaging of nuclei other than hydrogen has become more feasible. Four such applications are described in this chapter: diffusion, perfusion, functional imaging, and imaging of hyperpolarized noble gases.

12.1 Diffusion

As mentioned in Chapter 1, all matter is made of atoms, which bond to form molecules. These molecules continually move due to interactions with their surroundings. Two types of molecular movement can be observed in tissues. One is coherent bulk flow, which occurs for blood or cerebrospinal fluid. This movement arises from a difference in pressure between the two locations, produced by contractions of the heart. Direct visualization of blood flow within the vascular network is accomplished using MR angiographic techniques, as described in Chapter 11.

Another manifestation of this continuous movement of molecules is a relatively small (microscopic) random displacement of the molecule in space, known as Brownian motion. One of the most important examples in biological systems is diffusion. Diffusion of molecules occurs due to Brownian motion in the presence of a concentration difference between two regions, such as on either side of a cell membrane. Diffusion is a nonequilibrium thermodynamic process and is the process responsible for the random transport of gases and nutrients from the extracellular space into the cell interior. The molecular motion occurs from a region of high concentration to one of low concentration, analogous to heat flow between hot and cold regions. In pure solutions, diffusion is characterized by a constant known as the self-diffusion coefficient D, measured in units of $mm^2 \, s^{-1}$.

MRI Basic Principles and Applications, Fifth Edition.
Brian M. Dale, Mark A. Brown and Richard C. Semelka.
© 2015 John Wiley & Sons, Ltd. Published 2015 by John Wiley & Sons, Ltd.

Studies of diffusion in solutions have been performed using MR for many years. The standard method uses a symmetric pair of gradient pulses to increase the amount of spin dephasing observed in a spin echo (Figure 12.1). Known as the Stejskal–Tanner (Stejskal and Tanner, 1965) or the pulsed gradient spin echo (PGSE) method, spins that move during the gradient pulses experience unequal effects from the gradient pulses and do not rephase at the echo time *TE*. This causes a loss in signal amplitude from those spins:

$$S(TE, b) \propto \exp(-TE/T2) * \exp(-b * D) \qquad (12.1)$$

where *T*, *t*, and *G* are defined in Figure 12.1 and

$$b = \gamma^2 G^2 t^2 (T - t/3) \qquad (12.2)$$

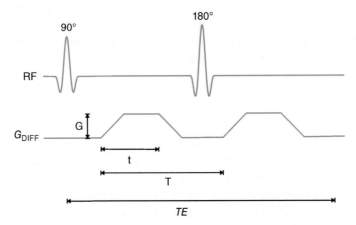

Figure 12.1 Spin echo pulse sequence showing diffusion gradients, known as the Stejskal – Tanner approach. *G* is the amplitude for each of the gradient pulses, *t* is the duration of the gradient pulse during which the diffusion weighting occurs, and *T* is the time between the two pulses.

The signal sensitivity to motion for the technique is determined by the "*b*" value. Larger *b* values can be obtained by using larger gradient amplitudes *G*, longer duration gradient pulses *t*, longer times between the gradient pulses *T*, additional gradient pulses, or combinations of all four. MRI applications of this technique are referred to as diffusion-weighted imaging. Solutions with small *D* values undergo little motion and sustain little signal loss in the image. Solutions with large *D* values move significantly during the gradient pulses and produce a significantly attenuated signal.

In biological systems, accurate measurements of diffusion in tissue are complicated by several factors:
1 Perfusional blood flow. Normal perfusion of tissue by flowing blood can be assessed through MR techniques as described below. However, blood flow through randomly oriented microscopic blood vessels within a tissue voxel results in a loss of signal, known as intravoxel incoherent motion or

"pseudodiffusion", which is indistinguishable from true diffusion. For this reason, measurements of diffusion in tissues *in vivo* measure a quantity known as the apparent diffusion coefficient (ADC), combining both sources of signal loss. The assumption is made that all signal loss is due to true diffusion and that the intravoxel incoherent motion is minimal.

2 *T2* effects. MRI measurements of diffusion are made using echo-based techniques with relatively long *TE* times (70 ms or longer), producing significant *T2* weighting in the images. Since diffusion also causes signal losses (see equation (12.1)), any measured signal loss from *T2* relaxation for a tissue could be confused with that caused by diffusion. In other words, signal changes in an image acquired with a large *b* and large *TE* may be caused by either tissues with a long *T2*, restricted water motion (small ADC), or both.

3 Directional dependence. In pure solutions, diffusion is isotropic in nature, meaning that *D* is equal in all directions. In tissues, the situation is more complicated. For many tissues, diffusion is anisotropic in nature, meaning that the ADC will have different values in different directions. In addition, the preferential directions for diffusion will generally not coincide with the gradient axes or with obvious patient anatomy; in other words, the sensitive directions for diffusion may not be readily apparent. Finally, diffusion in one direction may be significantly greater than in the other directions. A more accurate description for diffusion uses a mathematical notation known as a tensor, which represents the molecular motion as a 3×3 matrix.

The effects of intravoxel incoherent motion can be reduced by using high spatial resolution techniques to reduce the voxel size. However, this requires an increased scan time to achieve adequate SNR, which is often unacceptable, and it cannot be eliminated. However, in biological systems the intravoxel incoherent motion is usually significantly faster than diffusion, and so it can be eliminated by using higher diffusion encoding gradients or by modeling the signal loss as a biexponential function of the encoding strength.

To address *T2* effects, an ADC map may be calculated (Figure 12.2). This is an image, with pixel values corresponding to the ADC values for the tissue. Two or more images are acquired with different *b* values and the ADC value for a pixel is calculated based on equation (12.1) (substituting ADC for *D*). The range of *b* values is usually between 0 and 1000 s mm^{-2} or higher, with increased accuracy in estimating the ADC achieved using more *b* values. Low ADC values are characteristic of regions with restricted diffusion while regions where the spins are relatively free to move have high ADC values.

Two approaches are used to address the directional dependence of diffusion. The first approach is to acquire a trace image. This is an image created by averaging the diffusion in a voxel at a chosen *b* value in three directions. The trace image has the advantage that it is independent of the particular axes used for the measurement as long as they are orthogonal (perpendicular). In other words, the trace image is the same regardless of the gradient direction (invariant).

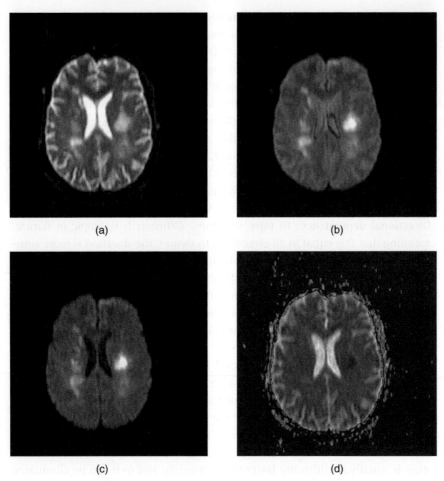

Figure 12.2 Diffusion-weighted EPI sequence: (a) b = 0 s mm^{-2}; (b) b = 500 s mm^{-2}; (c) b = 1000 s mm^{-2}. Normal tissue has moderate diffusion of water, while tissue under stress, such as that at risk for a stroke, has restricted motion of tissue water and shows increased signal on image with significant diffusion sensitivity. (d) ADC map, calculated from images (a), (b), and (c). Low pixel amplitudes indicate restricted water movement. High pixel amplitudes indicate free water movement.

This allows the three primary gradient axes (G_x, G_y, G_z) to be used. The trace images can provide an estimate of the amount of overall diffusion present in a tissue, but it discards the directional information available about molecular motion.

The other approach for analyzing the directional dependence is to measure the complete diffusion tensor and calculate the preferential directions for diffusion within the voxel. As mentioned above, the preferential directions for diffusion do not necessarily correspond to gradient directions nor macroscopic patient anatomy. To determine these directions, measurements are made with the two gradient pulses in Figure 12.1 having all possible gradient pairs $(G_x-G_x, G_x-G_y, G_x-G_z,$ etc.). The measurements made with the gradient directions in the same direction (e.g., G_x-G_x) will generate the diagonal elements of the tensor while those acquired with the gradient directions being different (e.g., G_x-G_y, G_x-G_z) will correspond to the nondiagonal terms of the tensor. Current measurement techniques allow for as many as 256 different gradient direction pairs to be made within a scan. The preferred direction(s) for diffusion can be determined by diagonalization of the tensor matrix (calculating the eigenvalues or characteristic values). The coordinate system that generates the diagonal representation for the tensor D_{DIAG} corresponds to the preferred diffusion directions (eigenvectors or principal axes). The eigenvalues correspond to the ADC along that particular direction.

Use of the eigenvector coordinate system to specify the diffusion directions is frequently used as it provides the simplest representation of diffusion. One common presentation is to display diffusion as a three-dimensional ellipsoid, with the axes of the ellipsoid representing the preferred diffusion directions, and the size of the ellipsoid in a given direction related to the square root of the eigenvalue (ADC) for that direction (Figure 12.3). Isotropic diffusion is represented as a sphere, with equal eigenvalues in all three directions and no preferred direction. Anisotropic diffusion will have one eigenvalue different from the other two or all three eigenvalues different. The first case will have an ellipsoid with two directions equal in length while the second case will have all three axes of different lengths. The principal diffusion direction is the axis with the largest ADC, represented as the longest dimension in the ellipsoid.

Another method of analysis of diffusion anisotropy divides the diffusion tensor into two parts, one describing the diffusion that is isotropic (D_{ISO}) and one containing the anisotropic component (D_{ANISO}). Two quantities can be derived from the anisotropic component. The relative anisotropy (RA) compares the magnitude of these two quantities:

$$RA = D_{ANISO}/D_{ISO} \tag{12.3}$$

while the fractional anisotropy (FA) compares the anisotropy to the diagonal representation:

$$FA = (3/2)^{1/2} * D_{ANISO}/D_{DIAG} \tag{12.4}$$

Both of these quantities are zero if diffusion is isotropic, but FA is used more frequently. Color is also used to represent the different components of the principal eigenvector (red $= x$ component; green $= y$ component; blue $= z$ component).

One of the most important applications of diffusion-weighted imaging is in the evaluation of cerebral ischemia and stroke. Normal cells maintain

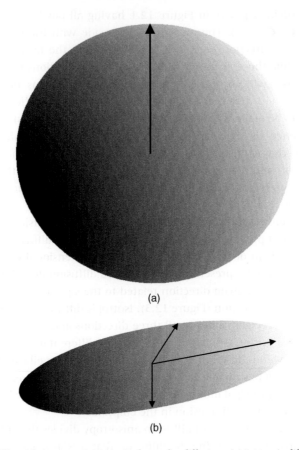

Figure 12.3 Ellipsoids representing principal axes for diffusion. (a) Isotropic diffusion: diffusion is equally likely in all directions and is represented by a sphere. (b) Anisotropic diffusion: diffusion is more likely in one or more directions. The direction that is most likely has the largest vector length.

a concentration gradient of sodium ions extracellular and potassium ions intracellular, and are surrounded by and contain water. The enzymatic process responsible for the maintenance of this gradient is known as active transport or the sodium–potassium–ATP pump. The energy for this process is provided by adenosine triphosphate (ATP), which in turn requires oxygen as one of the reactants for its production. The oxygen for this process is carried to the tissue from the lungs by erythrocytes as an O_2–hemoglobin coordination complex. Following the onset of ischemia and the loss of oxygen by the tissue, the ADC of the affected tissue water has been observed to decrease, leading to a decrease in signal dephasing and an increase in signal amplitude (see Figure 12.2). Although the reason for this decrease in ADC is unclear, it is presumably due to a change in the membrane permeability to the sodium and potassium ions and an accompanying increase in intracellular water content. This ADC decrease is reversible upon restoration of blood flow, provided it occurs before complete cell membrane breakdown.

12.2 Perfusion

Although angiographic techniques visualize the vascular network within a patient, they do not have sufficient spatial resolution to visualize blood flow through a tissue in bulk. However, it is possible in many instances to observe changes in tissue signal due to the blood flow through it, a process known as perfusion. Proper tissue perfusion is critical to ensure an adequate supply of nutrients to the constituent cells as well as removal of metabolic byproducts. It also aids in maintenance of a stable tissue temperature. Abnormalities in perfusion can lead to an increased temperature sensitivity and a loss of tissue viability through hypoxia.

 Three approaches are used for MR perfusion studies, two of which are analogous to radioisotope tracer studies and use similar methods for analysis of the flow dynamics. One approach acquires a series of rapid (less than 20 seconds per image) $T1$-weighted imaging studies following the bolus administration of a gadolinium-based contrast agent. These images are typically acquired using spoiled gradient echo, $T1$-weighted magnetization prepared or echo planar techniques. An increase in tissue signal occurs as the contrast agent infuses the extravascular spaces of the tissue. Perfusion defects are visualized as a lack of signal increase for the affected region of tissue. The other approach is useful if the contrast agent remains in the blood vessels, such as in cerebral tissue with an intact blood–brain barrier. In this case, the paramagnetic nature of the contrast agent increases the local tissue susceptibility, causing increased $T2^*$ dephasing of nearby tissues. Serial $T2^*$-weighted gradient echo or echo planar sequences are acquired, and the well-perfused tissue has a reduction of signal relative to the precontrast images or the poorly perfused tissues.

The third approach, known as arterial spin labeling (ASL), does not use contrast media to highlight the flowing spins. Instead, two sets of images are acquired, typically using an EPI pulse sequence. One set is acquired following an RF pulse that "tags" the spins outside the slice of interest, while the other set of images serves as a reference. Subtraction of the two images leaves an image of the tagged spins. A variable delay time between the tagging pulse and the data collection allows control of the tag position based on the flow velocity. Two approaches are frequently used. Pulsed arterial spin labeling (PASL) uses an inversion or saturation pulse that is either slice selective or nonselective to tag the moving spin. The tag may be applied to the moving spins or to the stationary tissue. Continuous arterial spin labeling (CASL) saturates the blood in one set of images, visualizing the blood in the reference image. Both methods are used to evaluate the hemodynamics in the tissue, most frequently the brain. The primary limitation to this approach is the limited SNR in the final images. Increased SAR is also a limitation.

Two examples where perfusion studies have shown promise are in the examination of abnormalities of blood flow within tissue and for the detection and characterization of tumors. Blood flow anomalies in the myocardium following infarction have been studied for many years using radionuclide agents. First-pass MR perfusion studies have shown good correlation with these studies and have enabled visualization of different phases of perfusion (Wilke et al., 1999). In these examinations, the measurement parameters are chosen so that the blood signal is minimal prior to contrast agent administration. Reduced uptake of the contrast agent in poorly perfused tissue causes a delay in signal enhancement. Liver studies following administration of gadolinium-based contrast agents have also demonstrated differences in tissue perfusion. Images acquired immediately following contrast administration show capillary phase perfusion, whereas images acquired 45 seconds postadministration show substantial portal phase

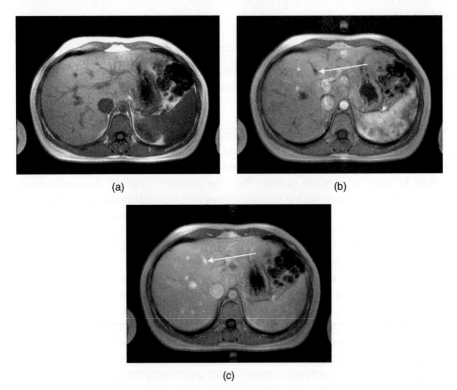

(a)   (b)

(c)

Figure 12.4 *T1*-weighted two-dimensional spoiled gradient echo imaging of liver following administration of gadolinium–chelate contrast agent. (a) Image acquired prior to contrast administration. (b) Image acquired immediately following administration. Contrast agent is in the hepatic arterial phase, as evidenced by the nonopacified hepatic vein (arrow). (c) Image acquired 45 seconds following administration. Contrast agent is now in the capillary phase, as evidenced by its presence in the hepatic vein (arrow).

perfusion (Figure 12.4). The normal spleen usually shows a serpigenous enhancement pattern immediately following contrast administration, with a more uniform signal intensity observed on images acquired 45 seconds or later.

The other studies where differential perfusion has been used are in the detection of certain tumors. Pituitary adenomas have demonstrated a difference in perfusion between microadenomas and macroadenomas following contrast administration (Finelli and Kaufman, 1993). Also, malignant breast tumors have demonstrated a significantly faster uptake of contrast media than benign tumors in some studies (Kvistad et al., 2000). Rapid scanning is necessary as both classes of tumors have similar signal amplitudes 3 minutes following contrast administration. Use of a 3D volume scan enables a bilateral breast study with good spatial and temporal resolution (Figure 12.5).

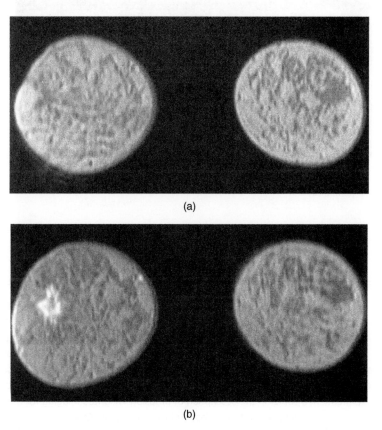

(a)

(b)

Figure 12.5 *T1*-weighted three-dimensional volume spoiled gradient echo imaging of breast following administration of gadolinium – chelate contrast agent. (a) Precontrast image, lacking evidence of lesion; (b – d) serial images acquired every 48 seconds following contrast agent administration. Note increased signal from lesion in later images.

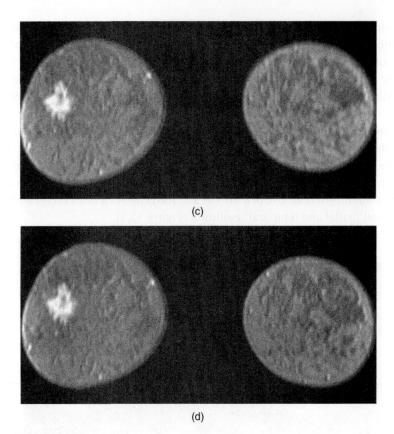

(c)

(d)

Figure 12.5 (*continued*)

12.3 Functional brain imaging

MRI can be used in the study of brain activity in response to an external stimulus. This is known as functional MRI (fMRI) to distinguish it from anatomical MRI. The basic approach is very similar to that mentioned earlier for bolus contrast agent studies of brain tissue, namely using $T2^*$-weighted gradient echo or echo planar images. However, instead of administering an exogenous agent to reduce the $T2^*$ relaxation time, the local tissue susceptibility is shortened by the presence of endogenous paramagnetic species present in blood. As mentioned earlier in the description of diffusion-weighted imaging for the evaluation of stroke, oxygen is delivered to cells bonded to hemoglobin. Oxygenated hemoglobin is diamagnetic, with a very small magnetic moment, while deoxygenated hemoglobin has a significant paramagnetic moment. Significant concentrations of deoxygenated hemoglobin shorten the $T2^*$ relaxation time of the tissue and result in a decrease in signal compared to tissue with oxygenated hemoglobin.

Brain activation studies are based on the assumption that stimulated tissue undergoes an increase in blood flow with an increased delivery of oxygenated hemoglobin. The amount of deoxygenated hemoglobin decreases within the tissue, reducing the concentration of para-magnetic molecules. This condition reduces the amount of susceptibility dephasing induced and thereby increases the $T2^*$ for the stimulated tissue relative to the unstimulated tissue. As a result, the stimulated tissue appears higher in signal on $T2^*$-weighted images. This phe-nomenon is known as the blood oxygenation level dependent effect or BOLD effect (DeYoe et al., 1994). The typical approach is to perform a large series of measurements in the presence and absence of the stimulus and statistically compare the images, identifying pixels presumably from the activated region of tissue.

Several aspects must be considered when performing BOLD fMRI studies. Correction for patient movement between measurements must be performed. Also, conversion to a standardized coordinate system is necessary if image comparison between patients (compensating for brain size, shape, and positional differences) and with other measurement techniques (CT, PET) is to be performed. The experimental paradigm or stimulus execution scheme is a critical aspect. Performance of the paradigm by the patient during the examination is of fundamental importance to ensure that the measured activation is a result of the executed paradigm. One approach used to confirm this correlation is to perform the measurements as several sets of paired scans (stimulus present, stimulus absent). The correlation coefficient of the voxel intensity and the time variation of the stimulus is also calculated to ensure that the observed variation is in response to the stimulus. A threshold of significance, known as the z score, must also be defined for the particular study below which the signal difference is assumed not to be relevant. Finally, the pixel intensity from the stimulated image typically exceeds that from the unstimulated image by less than 5%. This necessitates the repetition of the measurement many times (1000 or more) to ensure that the observed signal variation from the voxel is real and not artifactual in origin. High magnetic field strengths (1.5 T or greater) are necessary to increase the change in $T2^*$ between activated and nonactivated tissue. The development of scanners with B_0 of 3 T or greater have allowed more reliable and reproducible results to be obtained through an overall increase in SNR.

An important requirement for these examinations is a reproducible, stable performance of the scanner hardware. Deviations in hardware output should be less than 1% over 15 minutes or longer of continuous scanning. This requirement is much more stringent than is required for routine scanning. Environmental factors such as thermal stability of the scanner electronics and building vibrations are two common causes of abnormal signal variations in these examinations.

BOLD-type functional MRI studies have been used for studying many areas of the brain, including the visual, auditory, motor, and frontal cortex. Their results have compared favorably with those obtained using positron emission tomography (PET). Simple stimuli such as flashing lights or finger tapping have been used successfully. More complex stimuli such as cognitive processes (word or picture association) are currently being evaluated.

12.4 Ultra-high field imaging

Note that this section discusses concepts that are more fully explained in Chapter 14.

The development of MR scanners with B_0 significantly greater than 1.5 T presents a number of challenges. While clinically useful images have been demonstrated at field strengths of 7.0 T, commercially available clinical MRI systems are limited to 3.0 T or less. As of this writing, however, scanning at field strengths up to 8.0 T for subjects older than 1 month for research purposes is considered to be of low risk, subject to approval by local institutional review boards. The challenges of so-called ultra-high magnetic field scanners can be divided into two categories: those exclusive of patient tissue and those due to changes in the tissue response to the increased magnetic field.

As might be expected, many of the areas of concern with conventional field strength magnets are also valid with ultra-high field systems, and in some cases of greater concern. For example, current ultra-high field magnets are super-conducting solenoidal magnets and use liquid He as the cryogen, as are most conventional magnets. The higher field strengths require greater amounts of magnet wire windings, increasing the overall size and weight of the magnet, and greater amounts of electrical current to generate the magnetic field. The larger B_0 will also exert larger forces of attraction than conventional magnets of the same physical size. This will increase the audible noise of the scanner during measurements. The fringe magnetic field will also extend outside the magnet housing to a greater extent, increasing the influence of the environment on the magnet homogeneity. Shimming of the magnet is also more problematic, in that the absolute inhomogeneity (measured in Hz or μT over a particular distance or volume) increases with increased B_0 while the relative homogeneity (measured in ppm) might remain constant. Ferromagnetic objects must be kept at greater distances to prevent uncontrollable attraction into the bore. Safe distances for patients with metal implants or for electronic equipment will extend farther from the magnet isocenter. Proper site planning and preparation is critical for safe and successful magnet installations.

As with scanning at conventional B_0, there are issues with RF power at ultra-high field strengths. As stated in equation (1.1), the resonant frequency ω_0 is proportional to B_0. RF penetration is more difficult at higher frequencies, a phenomenon known as the skin effect. This can cause inhomogeneous excitation of a slice, producing shading in images. In addition, increased power from the transmitter is necessary to produce the RF pulses. As mentioned in Chapter 14, the power from a pulse is used in the calculation of the SAR for a scan. The power produced by a pulse is proportional to the square of its frequency, so that increasing B_0 by a factor of 2 increases the pulse power by a factor of 4. This means that whole-body scanning at ultra-high B_0 will require different examination protocols in order not to exceed the same SAR guidelines.

There are also tissue response differences to ultra-high B_0. The net magnetization M is directly proportional to B_0, so that the potential exists to obtain an increased signal. This is particularly beneficial for MR examinations of nuclei other than hydrogen. The absolute chemical shift difference between fat and water hydrogen atoms (measured in Hz) increases linearly with B_0, while it remains constant when measured in relative units (ppm). Increased receiver bandwidths will be required in order to reduce chemical shift artifacts to acceptable levels. On a practical basis, the maximum inherent SNR will increase proportionally to B_0. This can be exploited in two ways. Smaller voxels can be scanned allowing improved spatial resolution. For example, 1024×1024 image matrices with excellent image quality can be obtained with acceptable scan times using ETSE sequences. Alternately, MR scans can be acquired with equivalent SNR with fewer signal averages. This can result in shorter scans, allowing better time resolution in dynamic examinations.

There are additional tissue response issues that can have a significant effect on clinical scanning. As mentioned in Chapter 3, the $T1$ relaxation times increase significantly with increasing B_0 while the $T2$ relaxation times increase much less dramatically. This means that significant $T1$ saturation can occur in scans at ultra-high field strengths using measurement parameters that produce minimal saturation at conventional scanners. As a result, longer TR times are necessary to achieve equivalent tissue contrast. This aspect, together with the increased SAR, has limited use of traditional spin echo for acquiring $T1$ images of the brain or spine. Instead, use of gradient echo is being explored to provide acceptable image quality. There are also increased magnetic susceptibility differences at ultra-high B_0. This can produce more severe artifacts in areas where these differences are significant, but can be exploited when performing perfusion or functional MR examinations.

12.5 Noble gas imaging

As discussed in Chapter 1, the most common nucleus observed in MRI is ^{1}H, due to its high natural abundance and its large nuclear magnetic moment. In spite of these advantages, the net magnetization produced in patients by the ^{1}H atoms in water or fat through the Zeeman interaction at normal imaging magnetic fields is very small and induces a weak signal. Other attempts at measuring MR signals from endogenous nuclei such as ^{23}Na have succeeded, but their low sensitivity has limited their practical implementation.

Successful MRI studies of lung air spaces using hyperpolarized ^{3}He and ^{129}Xe gases have been reported (MacFall et al., 1996; Mugler et al., 1997). Visualizing lung air spaces using normal ^{1}H imaging is difficult due to low concentration of water in air, large magnetic susceptibility differences due to the paramagnetic nature of molecular oxygen, and artifacts from respiratory or cardiac motion.

Although the latter two problems can be minimized using rapid scan techniques with short *TE* times, the low signal amplitude produced by water vapor cannot. Helium and xenon are noble gases that are relatively unreactive and dissolve into tissues readily. They can rapidly permeate into the lung spaces. They are also well tolerated by most patients, with the most common side effect being a mild sedative effect produced by xenon.

The source of the MRI signal from noble gases is spin polarization between the parallel and antiparallel orientations, just as for any MR measurement, but it is generated in a different manner. Rather than using the natural thermal spin polarization produced by the MRI magnet, these gases are polarized outside the patient through the use of a laser and rubidium atoms. The rubidium atoms are excited by the laser and transfer the energy to the particular gas (^{3}He or ^{129}Xe). This results in a net magnetization 10,000–100,000 times that produced by the MRI magnet. This hyperpolarized gas is then inhaled by the patient through a ventilator bag. Gradient echo imaging techniques are used to produce images until the net magnetization is completely lost through *T2** relaxation (approximately one minute following inhalation) (Figure 12.6).

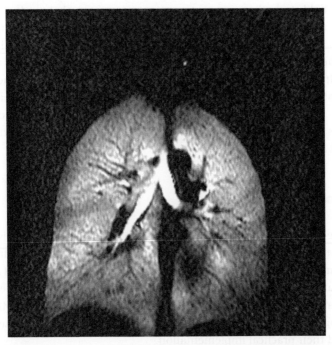

Figure 12.6 ^{3}He image of normal lung acquired following inhalation of hyperpolarized helium gas. Note significant signal in trachea and upper lobes of lungs and lack of signal from other tissue in the body. Measurement parameters: pulse sequence, two-dimensional refocused gradient echo, postexcitation; *TR*, 25 ms; *TE*, 10 ms; acquisition matrix, N_{PE}, 128 and N_{RO}, 256; FOV, 350 mm PE × 350 mm RO. (Reproduced with permission of James R. MacFall, Duke University.)

There are several technical difficulties in performing noble gas imaging. First, the ^{3}He and ^{129}Xe active isotopes are not the predominant isotopes for these nuclei (see Table 1.1). For this reason, they are relatively expensive and recovery of the gas following patient studies is performed to reduce the expense. Second, the resonant frequencies for these nuclei are very different from ^{1}H so that different transmitter and receiver coils are used from those used in standard MRI studies. Third, noble gas imaging is a single-pass study. Because of the method used to produce the net magnetization, there is no possibility for a repeat measurement following inhalation. Finally, only gradient echo techniques are possible. Spin echoes require 180° refocusing pulses and the recovery of net magnetization through *T1* relaxation prior to subsequent excitation pulses. There is no natural regeneration of the net magnetization of hyperpolarized noble gases once it is dephased.

CHAPTER 13

Magnetic resonance spectroscopy

Although MRI is the most common application of the MR phenomenon used in the medical community, it is a relatively recent development. The original application of magnetic resonance is MR spectroscopy (MRS), a technique that allows examination of individual molecules or portions of molecules within a sample. The development of whole-body scanners has allowed MRS to be used to study the biochemistry of disease processes within a patient without the need for invasive procedures such as biopsies. Many of the principles of MRS are the same as those of MRI, although their emphasis is somewhat different. While theoretically possible on any MRI system, most MRS studies are performed using magnets of 1.5 T or higher, due to the low intrinsic sensitivity of the technique. Hydrogen spectroscopic studies can be performed on standard imaging systems with no additional hardware required. Spectral studies of other nuclei require additional transmitter and receiver hardware (see Chapter 14). This chapter summarizes some of the basic concepts of hydrogen MRS. For more complete discussions of the field, see Salibi and Brown, 1998, Mukherji, 1998, and deGraaf, 2007.

13.1 Additional concepts

13.1.1 Chemical shift

A description of the basic principles of MRS begins at the same place as that of a description of the principles of MRI. The basic concepts of net magnetization produced by a collection of spins in a magnetic field, signal production following absorption of RF energy, and $T1$ and $T2$ relaxation as described in Chapters 1 through 3 are identical for MRS and MRI. However, there are two important differences between MRS and MRI. First, MRS signals are normally detected in the absence of a gradient. All molecules are detected in the presence of the same base magnetic field. The chemical shift described in Chapter 2 is the only source of magnetic field variation present during signal detection. Rather than be the source of an artifactual signal as it is in MRI, the chemical shift is the means by which molecular species are identified in MRS studies. Second, unlike MRI, relaxation effects are avoided as much as possible in

MRI Basic Principles and Applications, Fifth Edition.
Brian M. Dale, Mark A. Brown and Richard C. Semelka.
© 2015 John Wiley & Sons, Ltd. Published 2015 by John Wiley & Sons, Ltd.

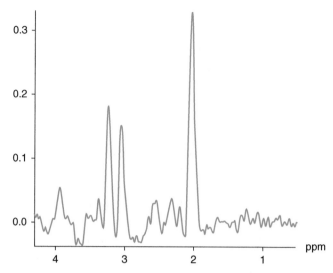

Figure 13.1 Typical ^{1}H spectrum from normal brain. Measurement parameters: pulse sequence, two-dimensional CSI PRESS; *TR*, 1500 ms; *TE*, 144 ms; N_{SA}, 4; voxel size, $10 \times 10 \times 15$ mm^3.

MRS studies. The molecules under observation are relatively small in size and have relatively long *T1* and *T2* values. Long *TR* (typically $\geq$ 1500 ms) are used in order to minimize *T1* saturation effects as well as allowing for high-frequency resolution. *T2* dephasing effects are dominated by main field inhomogeneities and are more properly described by *T2**.

As mentioned in Chapter 2, chemical shift values are measured to a reference frequency. The traditional reference frequency used for ^{1}H is that of tetramethyl-silane (TMS). This is impractical to use in biological systems due to its toxicity and the difficulty in achieving uniform tissue distribution. In its place, an endogenous secondary reference is normally used. This is the methyl ^{1}H signal of *N*-acetyl aspartate, which has a chemical shift of 2.0 ppm relative to TMS. This allows standard tables of chemical shifts to be used and for *in vivo* spectral displays to correlate with traditional *ex vivo* displays (Figure 13.1).

MRS is one application where the use of increased field strengths will cause the spectral appearance to change. As mentioned previously in Chapter 2, the chemical shift is a relative scale and the chemical shift values are independent of frequency. However, the individual signals and their absolute frequencies increase with increased field strength. This concept was presented in the context of fat and water ^{1}H frequency differences and the chemical shift artifact, though this principle is true for all signals. The typical *in vivo* spectral display ranges from 0.0 to 4.5 ppm, which is characteristic of ^{1}H atoms that are part of CH$_3$–, CH$_2$–, or CH– functional groups. This 4.5 ppm range of frequencies corresponds to approximately 285 Hz at 1.5 T, while it spans 570 Hz at 3.0 T. The resonance linewidths (see below) are normally dominated by magnetic field inhomogeneities, which can be reduced through shimming. If the linewidth is equal in Hz at the two field strengths, then the peaks of the higher field spectra will appear sharper and better resolved.

The chemical shift provides the means by which portions of molecules are identified. The difference in ω is caused by differences in the local magnetic environment around the nucleus. This difference arises primarily from the electrons surrounding the nucleus (producing chemical shielding) and the atoms that are either bonded to or near the spins under observation. Because many molecules have similar chemical structures and the molecular differences may not be near the spins under observation, different molecules may have very similar spectra. For example, creatine and phosphocreatine differ chemically by the presence of a phosphate group in place of a hydrogen atom (Figure 13.2). However, the methyl portion of the molecule is the same and the MR signal from that functional group will be the same in both molecules. In a similar fashion, fatty acids with long hydrocarbon chains will have very similar spectra. Because of this, MRS studies are considered to be very sensitive techniques to detect the presence of a functional group but not specific enough to uniquely identify the molecule to which it is attached.

13.1.2 Spin coupling

In addition to the chemical shift, there is another molecular interaction that modifies the environment of a spin. Spins located on the same or adjacent atoms in a molecule interact with each other and each has its local magnetic field affected. The most common instance of this in biological systems is facilitated by the bonding electrons in the molecule and is known as spin coupling or J coupling. Spin coupling differs from the chemical shift in two very important ways: it is independent of magnetic field strength (chemical shifts increase with B_0 when measured in Hz) and there is always another spin involved in the coupling. First-order coupling occurs when the chemical shift difference is large relative to J:

$$\Delta\omega \geq 10\,J_{AX} \tag{13.1}$$

where J_{AX} is the coupling constant between spins A and X. Second-order coupling occurs when equation 13.1 is not met.

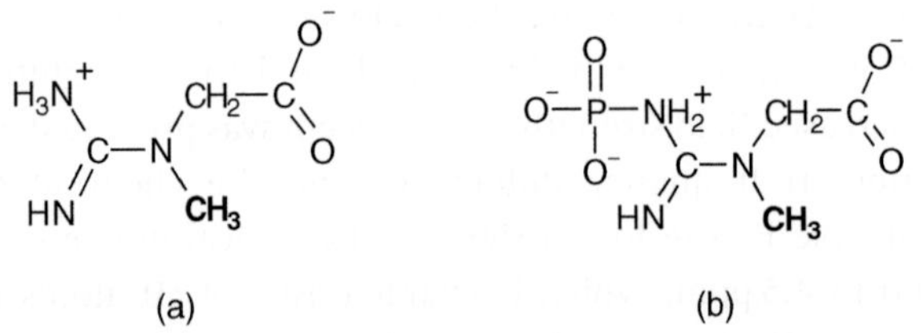

(a)   (b)

Figure 13.2 Chemical structures of creatine (a) and phosphocreatine (b). Because the phosphate group is located several bonds away, it has very little influence on the molecular environment of the methyl hydrogens (boldface type). As a result, the signals for the methyl hydrogens in both molecules have the same frequency.

Spin coupling involves a pairing interaction between spins on the same molecule that causes the MR signal of each member to be divided. The number of resultant signals and their relative amplitudes depend on the number of spins of each type. For hydrogen MRS studies in biological systems, the molecule where spin coupling is most easily viewed is lactate, $CH_3\underline{C}HOHCOO^-$. Attached to the middle carbon of the molecule (indicated by the underline) is a methyl group and a hydrogen atom. The hydrogen atom can be oriented parallel or antiparallel to B_0. The methyl group will sense slightly different molecular magnetic fields in each case. On average, there will be an equal number of possibilities for the hydrogen atom in each orientation, so the signal detected for the methyl group is split into two peaks separated by approximately 7 Hz, centered around the chemical shift for the methyl group. The 7 Hz value is the coupling constant J for this particular interaction between this set of spins. In a similar fashion, the methyl protons can be arranged in one of four configurations: all three parallel to B_0, all three antiparallel to B_0, two parallel and one antiparallel to B_0, or one parallel and two antiparallel to B_0. The last two configurations occur three times more frequently than the first two, so that the hydrogen atom will be divided into four peaks with relative amplitudes 1:3:3:1, each separated by 7 Hz. Because of its low amplitude and its nearness to the water resonant frequency, this resonance is normally not visualized in *in vivo* MRS studies.

An important feature of spin coupling is that it is not reversed by the application of a 180° refocusing RF pulse. As discussed below, one method of spatial localization uses 180° refocusing RF pulses to produce a spin echo. The lactate signal is modulated in amplitude, based on the elapsed time between the RF pulses, which means that the lactate protons may or may not be in phase with the other protons at the echo time TE. This condition is analogous to the phase modulation seen in gradient echo MRI studies for fat and water. The rate of this modulation is proportional to $1/J$. For the 7 Hz coupling, it corresponds to a phase modulation period of approximately 288 ms. Use of a TE of 288 ms ensures that the lactate resonances are in phase with the other noncoupled resonances, while use of a TE of 144 ms has the lactate signals 180° out of phase compared to the other resonances (Figure 13.3).

13.1.3 Spectral linewidth

The signals emitted by the spins will not be a single frequency line but will be a peak (or peaks if spin coupling is present) with a finite linewidth centered at the frequency corresponding to the chemical shift, as seen in Figures 13.1 and 13.3. The width of the peak, known as the full-width at half-maximum height (FWHM), is proportional to $1/T2*$:

$$FWHM \propto 1/T2* \tag{13.2}$$

As a result, the linewidth will change, depending on the particular molecule as well as the magnet homogeneity or shim. For signals with chemical shifts that

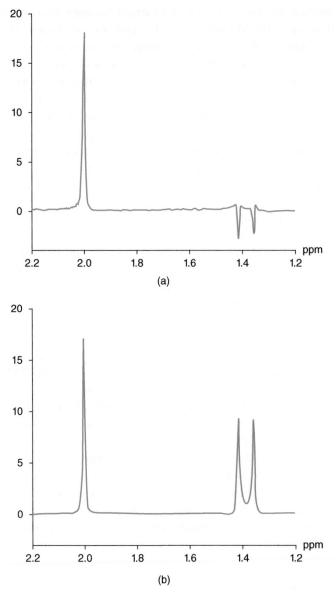

Figure 13.3 PRESS ^{1}H spectra of lactate (doublet) and acetate (singlet). Choice of *TE* affects the relative polarity of lactate peak compared to acetate, due to modulation of spin-coupled ^{1}H atoms. (a) *TE* = 144 ms; (b) *TE* = 288 ms.

are similar in value, such as creatine/phosphocreatine (Cr, 3.0 ppm) and choline (Cho, 3.2 ppm), the magnet homogeneity must be very high to adequately resolve the signals. This makes MRS examinations difficult in areas where significant magnetic susceptibility differences are present, such as the posterior fossa or near the skull.

In addition, the spectral or frequency resolution must be sufficiently high so that there are several data points defining the peak. For example, to resolve Cr and Cho, separated by 0.2 ppm (12 Hz at 1.5 T, 24 Hz at 3.0 T), a frequency resolution of approximately 1 Hz per point is typically used with a total frequency range of 1000 Hz acquired. To achieve this resolution, dwell times of 1 ms per point are required with the resulting total sampling time being 1 second or longer.

13.1.4 Water suppression

Clinical MRI techniques visualize the water and fat within the desired slice. The high concentration of water and fat within the tissue makes this feasible. In MRS, the metabolites under observation are as much as 10,000 times less concentrated than water, which makes their detection in the presence of tissue water difficult. In order to accomplish this, suppression of the water is necessary. The most common approach uses a frequency-selective RF pulse or pulses centered at the water resonant frequency to saturate the water protons. This technique is analogous to the fat saturation pulse described in Chapter 7. Water suppression factors of 100 or more are possible from a single pulse, making it an easy and effective way for reducing the signal contamination from water.

13.2 Localization techniques

Current techniques used for spatial localization of the MRS signals were derived from similar techniques used in MRI. Slice-selective excitation pulses in conjunction with gradient pulses are used to localize the RF energy to the desired volume of tissue, in the same manner as described in Chapter 4. However, unlike MRI, where the voxel size is typically $1 \times 1 \times 5$ mm^3 or less, MRS voxel sizes are usually $15 \times 15 \times 15$ mm^3 or larger. Therefore, MRS studies are limited to the examination of relatively large regions of tissue. The two general categories of localization techniques are based on the number of separate voxels from which spectra are obtained in each measurement.

13.2.1 Single voxel techniques

Single voxel techniques (also called single voxel spectroscopy, or SVS) acquire spectra from a single small volume of tissue. The most common approaches excite only the desired tissue volume through the intersection of three RF excitation pulses. Two schemes of RF pulsing are used. The first approach, known as point resolved spectroscopy (PRESS), uses a 90° and two 180° RF pulses in a fashion similar to a standard multiecho sequence (Figure 13.4). Each RF pulse is applied using a different physical gradient as the slice selection gradient. Only protons located at the intersection of all three pulses produce the spin echo at the desired *TE*. The other approach, known as the stimulated echo acquisition

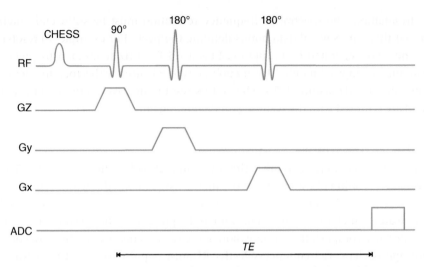

Figure 13.4 PRESS pulse sequence timing diagram. The CHESS RF pulse is used for suppression of water.

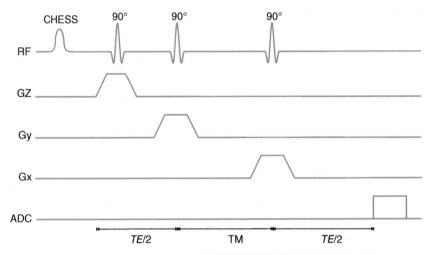

Figure 13.5 STEAM pulse sequence timing diagram. The CHESS RF pulse is used for suppression of water.

method (STEAM), uses three 90° RF pulses, each with a different slice selection gradient (Figure 13.5). The resulting stimulated echo (see Section 9.2.5, Coherence artifacts) is produced by protons located at the intersection of the pulses.

There are several differences between PRESS and STEAM. The major difference is in the nature of the echo signal. In PRESS, the entire net magnetization from the voxel is refocused to produce the echo signal; in STEAM, a maximum of one-half of the entire net magnetization generates the stimulated echo. As a result, PRESS has an SNR significantly larger than for STEAM for equivalent scan parameters. Another difference is that PRESS uses 180° RF pulses while STEAM uses only 90° RF pulses. The voxel dimensions with PRESS may be limited by the high transmitter power required for the 180° RF pulses. STEAM spectra are also unaffected by J coupling of spins, while PRESS spectra show a modulation of the signal from any coupled spins, such as lactate methyl protons. Finally, STEAM allows for shorter TE values, reducing signal losses from $T2$ relaxation and allowing observation of metabolites with short $T2^*$.

13.2.2 Multiple voxel techniques

Multiple voxel techniques are those from which multiple spectra are obtained during a single measurement. The most common of these methods is known as chemical shift imaging (CSI). CSI techniques are analogous to standard imaging techniques in that phase encoding gradient tables are used for spatial localization. They are subdivided into 1D, 2D, and 3D versions, depending on the number of gradient tables used for spatial localization. The most common of these approaches is two-dimensional CSI, in which two gradient tables are used. Volume-selective RF excitation pulses are used, either with a PRESS or STEAM RF pulse train. The most common scheme has the three excitation pulses in mutually perpendicular directions and is termed volume-selective CSI (Figure 13.6). This scheme enables the volume of excitation to be tailored so that areas producing a contaminating signal can be avoided. For example, brain studies using volume-selective CSI can minimize the signal from the skull and subcutaneous fat.

Volume-selective CSI techniques have the advantage over SVS techniques in that spectra from several volumes of tissue can be measured simultaneously, which is advantageous if the disease under observation is diffuse or covers a large area of anatomy. However, the measurement times for CSI techniques are generally relatively long and the entire data collection must be completed in order to obtain all the localization phase encoding steps. With SVS techniques, the measurement times are long due to multiple acquisitions necessary to produce adequate SNR, but the number of acquisitions can be adjusted depending on the voxel size. In addition, the multiple voxels must be individually postprocessed, making analysis of CSI data more operator intensive.

13.3 Spectral analysis and postprocessing

The MRS signal from a voxel contains information regarding the identity, molecular environment, and concentration of the metabolite producing the signal. This information is provided by the resonant frequency, the linewidth, and the integrated peak area, respectively. Although this information can be extracted from the time domain form of the signal, it is more convenient to analyze the frequency domain form, obtained following a Fourier transformation. This analysis

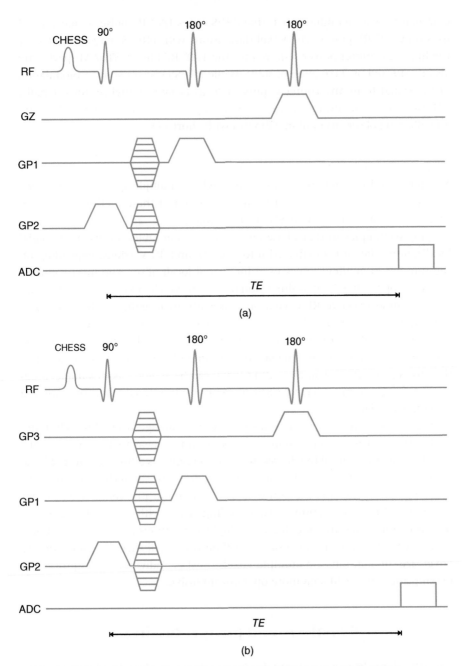

Figure 13.6 Volume-selective pulse sequence timing diagrams: (a) two-dimensional; (b) three-dimensional. The CHESS RF pulse is used for suppression of water.

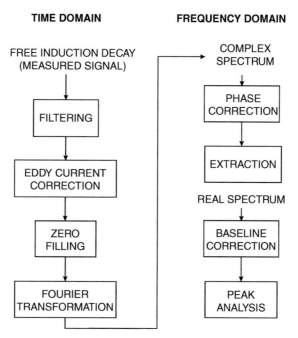

Figure 13.7 Typical spectroscopy postprocessing steps.

is aided by various data processing techniques applied both prior to and following the Fourier transformation (Figure 13.7). Many of these techniques are often used in MRI. Filtering of the echo signal is performed to reduce noise that can be induced during the very long sampling times for the signal. This is the same type of filter used in MRI to reduce truncation artifacts. Zero filling consists of adding data points of zero amplitude to the end of the detected time domain signal. In most cases, the extra points are appended to the end of the sampled data. These data are typically background noise in the measurement. Following Fourier transformation, the frequency resolution of the resulting spectrum is increased through interpolation of the measured data points. This approach, termed sinc interpolation in MRI, provides a smoother appearance to the final spectrum. The final processing that is applied to the time domain signal is a correction for distortion by residual eddy currents. Eddy currents are produced as a result of the time-varying nature of the gradient pulses and result in fluctuating magnetic fields that distort the MR signal. Manufacturers incorporate some type of eddy current compensation in the scanner hardware to correct for this, as described in Chapter 14. While sufficient for MRI studies, this compensation is seldom adequate to produce distortion-free MR spectra. Acquisition of a second signal, usually a water-unsuppressed signal from the same voxel, is used to provide a reference for residual field variations due to eddy currents. Alternately, if the eddy currents are not too severe, a small amount of water signal may be retained and can be used as the reference signal.

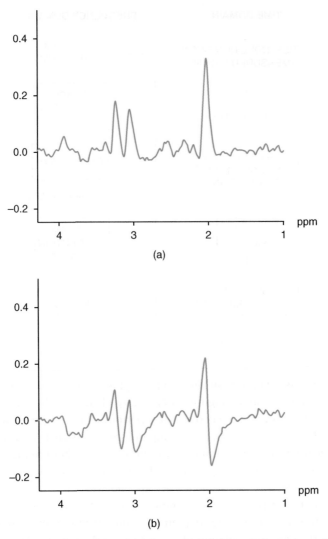

Figure 13.8 Phase-corrected complex spectrum resulting from Fourier transformation of FID signal. (a) Real portion of spectrum, also known as the absorption spectrum; (b) imaginary portion of spectrum, also known as the dispersion spectrum.

Following Fourier transformation, the resulting complex frequency domain signal is not a single mode signal, but is usually a mixture of both the in-phase (dispersion) and out-of-phase (absorption) signals relative to the transmitter (Figure 13.8). In MRI studies, rather than separating these two signals, they are combined to form the magnitude image. For MRS studies, the pure absorption mode is preferred, due to its simpler spectra and narrower linewidths, and to enable semiquantitative spectral analysis. A process known as phase correction is used to separate the two modes and extract the absorption portion. A mathematical manipulation combines the two components of the complex signal together in such a way as to isolate the absorption mode to the real portion and the dispersion mode to the imaginary portion. For the real spectrum, it may also be necessary to perform a baseline correction if it is not flat due to hardware imperfections or incomplete water suppression. Finally, the resonant frequency, linewidth, and integrated area for each peak in the spectrum can be measured. Although a visual examination of the spectrum can provide an approximation of these parameters, the most accurate method for analysis involved fitting of the peaks to theoretical curves of the appropriate lineshape. Whereas the frequencies and linewidths can be compared directly from one spectrum to another, peak areas are influenced by various hardware-related variables that are difficult to quantify. Instead, ratios of peak areas are used in evaluating the relative concentrations of the metabolites. Absolute concentrations for metabolites can be determined if a simultaneous measurement of a reference compound is performed in which the concentration of the reference is known by other means.

It is important to establish standardized scan protocols and to become familiar with the spectra from given anatomical regions as well as age-related variations. Peak patterns can vary so that an abnormal spectrum in one region is actually normal for another one (Figure 13.9a to c).

One example of a clinical application of MRS is in the evaluation of temporal lobe epilepsy. Normal brain spectra obtained with long TE (135 and 270 ms) show three major peaks: N-acetyl aspartate (NAA) at 2.0 ppm, Cr at 3.0 ppm, and Cho at 3.2 ppm relative to water at 4.7 ppm. The relative area ratios in adults are typically 1.4–1.5 for NAA/Cr and 0.8 for Cho/Cr. Patients with temporal lobe epilepsy have been found to have reduced levels of NAA and increased levels of Cho and Cr in the diseased lobe (Achten et al., 1997). Acquisition of spectra from both temporal lobes enables a clear identification of the affected region.

Another example is in the grading of gliomas through the presence of myo-Inositol (mIno), which has a resonance at 3.6 ppm corresponding to a methine group and can be observed using short TE acquisitions. High-grade versus low-grade gliomas have been distinguished by examining the Cho/Cr ratios as well as mIno/Cr ratios (Pinker et al., 2012).

A final example is in the assessment of prostate cancer. Normal prostate spectra show signals from the CH_3 of citrate at 2.6 ppm (Figure 13.10) as well as from Cho. Malignant tissue shows a significantly reduced citrate signal relative to Cho (Pinker et al., 2012). Prostate studies are challenging for several reasons. Frequently an endorectal surface coil is used. The small size and limited observation field of the coil make accurate placement a necessity. Use of torso array coils reduce the SNR, but provide for better patient cooperation.

13.4 Ultra-high field spectroscopy

MRS examinations also benefit from use of ultra-high B_0. As mentioned in Chapter 1, the net magnetization M is directly proportional to B_0, so that the

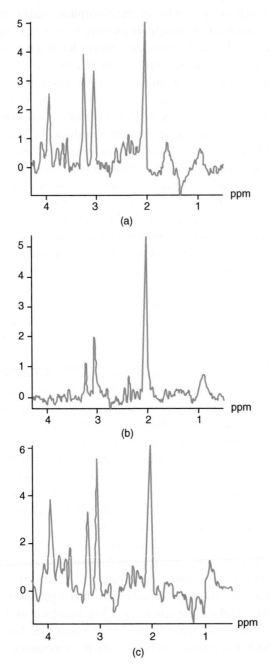

Figure 13.9 ^{1}H two-dimensional CSI PRESS spectra from different voxel locations. Note the difference in spectral patterns.

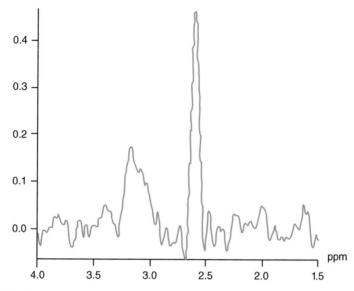

Figure 13.10 Normal prostate spectra.

potential exists to obtain an increased signal. This is particularly beneficial for MRS examinations of ^{31}P and ^{13}C, where the sensitivity is significantly less than that of ^{1}H (see Table 1.1). The increased chemical shift difference enables better spectral resolution between metabolites with similar resonant frequencies. The spectral linewidths generally appear narrower, due to the increased absolute frequency range that is displayed. On a practical basis, the increased SNR can be exploited in two ways. Smaller voxels can be scanned, allowing improved spatial resolution. For example, MR spectra can be acquired with an equivalent SNR with fewer signal averages. This can result in shorter scan times, allowing better time resolution in kinetic examinations. Alternately, resolution of gray and white matter into separate voxels can be performed using two-dimensional CSI (Figure 13.11).

There are two areas where ultra-high B_0 can cause problems. The signal from fat will significantly increase compared to that measured at conventional B_0. Suborbital fat or fat from bone marrow in the skull can potentially cause contamination in brain examinations. Outer volume saturation or narrow-band inversion of the lipid signal may be necessary to obtain good quality spectra. The second area of concern is due to the increased chemical shift differences between metabolite signals. When using volume-selective excitation, there will be a misregistration of the metabolites being excited by the frequency-selective RF pulse. Specifically, RF pulses broadcast at a given frequency will excite water protons at one location but metabolites at different locations. This is analogous to the chemical shift artifact observed in MRI. In particular, this is problematic with two-dimensional CSI, where the excitation volume is localized in all

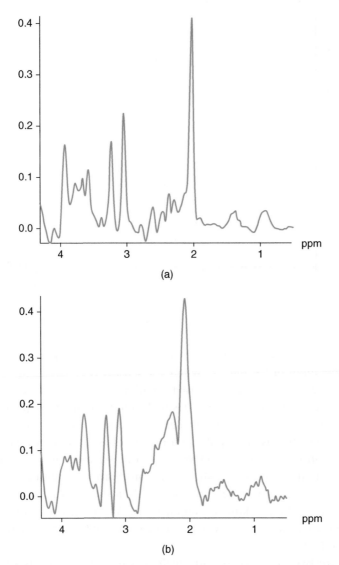

Figure 13.11 ^{1}H two-dimensional CSI PRESS spectra acquired at 1.5 T (a) and 3.0 T (b). The scan parameters are identical except that spectrum (a) had four averages, whereas spectrum (b) had one average.

three directions by frequency-selective RF pulses. Voxels near the edges of the excitation volume will exhibit intensity variations due to nonuniform metabolite excitation. While this problem is observed at conventional B_0, it is worsened at ultra-high B_0 due to the increased chemical shift between the metabolite resonances. Care must be taken in positioning the excitation volume as a result.

CHAPTER 14

Instrumentation

A very important aspect of the production of MRI images is the instrumentation used in the measurement. Many MR systems are commercially available, each possessing different features and capabilities that are often difficult to evaluate and compare objectively. Many of these features are based on the operating software provided by the manufacturer, but certain hardware components are common to all systems. The following sections describe the basic subsystems of an MRI scanner and technical aspects to consider when comparing scanners from different manufacturers. The major components are a computer system, a magnet system, a gradient system, a radiofrequency system, and a data acquisition system (Figure 14.1).

14.1 Computer systems

From its very origin, MRI has been a computer-driven technology. Over the last 30 years, as computers have increased in speed and capabilities, MRI scanners have taken advantage of this performance increase to become less hardware-intensive and more software-driven. This has allowed manufacturers to provide products that are more reliable and stable in hardware performance and more robust and flexible in the types of images that can be acquired.

There are three primary tasks performed on an MR scanner that are computer-based: general scanner control (user interface), image processing, and data collection (measurement control). Depending on the particular manufacturer, there may be one, two, or three computers that are present. The main or host computer controls the user interface software. It will be connected to a keyboard and one or more monitors for displaying images and text information, known as the console. The operating software for the main console enables the operator to control all functions of the scanner, either directly or indirectly. Scan parameters may be selected or modified, patient images may be displayed or recorded on film or other media, and postprocessing such as region-of-interest measurements or magnification can be performed. Several peripheral devices are typically attached to the main computer. One or more hard disks are used to

MRI Basic Principles and Applications, Fifth Edition.
Brian M. Dale, Mark A. Brown and Richard C. Semelka.
© 2015 John Wiley & Sons, Ltd. Published 2015 by John Wiley & Sons, Ltd.

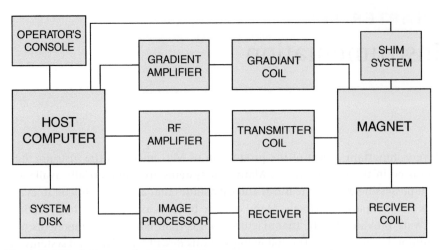

Figure 14.1 Block diagram of an MRI system.

store the patient images immediately following reconstruction. This disk or disks are used for short-term storage, with current disk drives able to store upwards of hundreds of thousands to millions of images, depending on the image size. A device for long-term archival storage, either CD or DVD, is usually included. A hard-copy camera may be connected via a network.

The image processing computer is used for performing the Fourier transformations or other processing of the detected data. This computer is synchronized with the host computer and the measurement controller. The raw data generated during the scan is stored from the receiver into memory in the image processor itself or on to a separate hard disk. Current image processing computers have multiple processors, either central processing units or graphical processing units, which allow for data processing in parallel, providing added speed in image reconstruction.

The third computer is the measurement controller, which interprets the operator-defined scan parameters and pulse sequence template files to generate the RF and gradient waveforms used to manipulate the spins. It also may be used as the monitor of the hardware to ensure its proper operation. This computer may be a separate processor or its functionality may be performed by one of the other two computers mentioned previously.

Additional consoles may be directly attached to the main computer, allowing convenient viewing or postprocessing of the images. More frequently, other viewing stations may be completely detached from the primary computer system and access the image data through a network connection. They may be used as a common viewing station for analysis of images from additional imaging modalities such as computed tomography, ultrasound, or traditional X-ray. In addition, there may be an archive server known as a PACS (picture archiving and communications system) unit. This system is used as a centralized digital repository for images. PACSs allow multiple users to access the images and patient data easily and can provide long-term archiving of the images in a central location.

MRI systems are most frequently incorporated into a computer network for the imaging facility. This allows images to be transferred directly from the MRI host computer to another computer in a remote location rather than using a removable medium (e.g., a CD). The interconnection between the two computers is normally a high-speed Ethernet connection. This is typically used for connecting computers within a local area network, typically consisting of a single building or small group of buildings; for example, between two scanners or between the scanner and a viewing station. This local network is often connected to the Internet, which is used for long-distance transmission of images and data.

Most computer networks use a communications protocol known as TCP/IP (Transmission Control Protocol/Internet Protocol) for the actual data transfer between the computers. Each computer on the network will have a unique identification number assigned to it by the network administrator, known as the IP address. This is a series of four numbers, each less than 256, (written as, for example, 121.232.22.21), which act as an electronic "street address" for the computer on the network. There will also be one computer or device on the network known as a router, which facilitates the data transfer. Data transfer is initiated from one computer (e.g., the MRI host computer) with the IP address of the destination computer (e.g., viewing station). The data are initially sent to the router, which will direct the data to the destination computer based on the IP address. Both the initiating and destination computers must have each other's IP address in order to transfer data in both directions.

While the usage of TCP/IP provides a means for transferring data between computers, there must be a common format (similar to a language) for writing the data if it is to be interpreted correctly. This is of particular importance if the two computers use software from different manufacturers, as each manufacturer will use their own proprietary format for data storage. One format that has become the industry standard for image and medical data transfer to facilitate such transfer is known as DICOM, which stands for Digital Imaging and Communications in Medicine. It is the result of a joint committee of the American College of Radiology and the National Electrical Manufacturers Association (ACR-NEMA). The DICOM standard provides a framework that allows equipment (scanners, digital cameras, viewing stations) from different manufacturers to accept and process data accurately. Images written using this standard have the basic measurement information stored so that any vendor can read and properly display the images with the correct anatomic labeling and basic measurement parameters. Manufacturers who subscribe to the DICOM standard have available a DICOM Conformance Statement, which provides details on their implementation. Programmers writing software that use DICOM-formatted images should consult the Conformance Statement for the particular manufacturer to ensure proper interpretation of the image header variables.

While a discussion of the complete DICOM standard is beyond the scope of the current discussion, two aspects of it are likely to be encountered with current MRI systems. The first is the format in which images are stored. Images stored using the DICOM format are written with the measurement parameters and other information organized in a fashion as specified in the DICOM Conformance Statement. This allows image display and analysis programs to be written without knowledge of the manufacturer's proprietary methods. Programs for reading, manipulating, and displaying DICOM-format images are available from several companies, with some programs available for free while others available for a fee.

The second aspect of DICOM that is frequently encountered is in the nature of the data transfer between computers. The DICOM standard has features that control the communication relationship between systems. This is critical to ensure confidentiality of patient information. Four communication protocols are commonly used. The first protocol controls the data transfer between a scanner and a hard-copy device, such as a laser camera. It is known as DICOM Basic_Print. This protocol enables the camera to be detached from the scanner, yet receive and process the image data over the computer network. Two other protocols control data transfer between workstations or a scanner. These work in tandem, known as the DICOM Service Class User and Service Class Provider (commonly known as Send/Receive). These protocols allow one computer system (e.g., a scanner) to send images to another system or to receive images from another system. This is normally used to connect scanners of different modalities (i.e., MR to CT). The other level of connectivity is known as the DICOM Query Service Class (commonly known as Query/Retrieve). This allows a remote computer to query the image database on a scanner and retrieve the images without requiring operator intervention. This is the normal connectivity between two scanners of the same modality or between a scanner and a PACS server. The DICOM connectivity is controlled by the Application Entity Title (AET) and both computers must have matching AETs in order for the transfer to be successful. The connectivity relationships are assigned by the network administrator during system installation or configuration based on the preferences and policies of the facility.

14.2 Magnet system

The magnet is the basic component of an MRI scanner. Magnets are available in a variety of field strengths, shapes, and materials. All magnet field strengths are measured in units of tesla or gauss (1 tesla = 10, 000 gauss). Magnets are usually categorized as low-, medium-, or high-field systems. Although the categorization is not fixed, low-field magnets are usually considered to be magnets that have B_0 less than 0.5 T. Medium-field systems have B_0 between 0.5 T and 1.5 T, high-field systems have fields between 1.5 T and 3.0 T, and ultra-high-field systems have B_0 greater than 3.0 T. The magnetic field is one area where caution should be exercised. Refer to Chapter 16 for a description of safety issues regarding the magnetic field.

Magnets are also characterized by the metal used in their composition. Permanent magnets are manufactured from metal that remains magnetic for extremely long periods of time (years). They can be solenoidal (tube shaped) or have a more open design such as a C-arm or double-doughnut. Permanent magnets have minimum maintenance costs because the field is always present. However, care must be taken to keep ferromagnetic material away from the magnet. Such material will be attracted forcefully into the magnet and the magnetic field cannot be turned off to allow its extraction. Permanent magnets also have their mass concentrated over a small area. Additional structural support of the scan room may be necessary in some situations. The scan room temperature must also be very stable as fluctuations in the temperature of the magnet metal will cause the field strength to change.

The other types of magnet are electromagnets in which the flow of electrical current through wire coils produces the magnetic field (current flowing through a wire generates a magnetic field perpendicular to the direction of the current flow). The magnetic field is present as long as current flows through the magnet windings. Traditional electromagnets are made of copper wire wound in loops of various shapes. They may be also solenoidal or open-type design. A power supply provides a constant current source. Due to the limited amount of current that copper wire can carry, copper wire-based electromagnets are low-field systems. They are also sensitive to room temperature variations.

The most common type of magnets are solenoidal electromagnets using niobium–titanium alloy wire immersed in liquid helium as the magnet wire. This alloy, which has the property known as superconductivity, has no resistance to the flow of electrical current below a temperature of 20 K. It also is capable of carrying large amounts of current, enabling high magnetic field strengths to be achieved. The magnet cryostat, which contains the liquid helium, may be a double dewar design with a liquid nitrogen container surrounding the helium container or a helium-only design with a refrigeration system to reduce the helium boiloff. Refrigeration systems used with current magnets allow essentially zero helium boiloff in the course of normal operation. The cryostat and helium reservoir insulates the magnet wire so that the magnetic field is very stable and less sensitive to room temperature fluctuations. Cryogens are a second area where caution should be exercised. Refer to Chapter 16 for a description of safety issues regarding the presence of cryogens.

 The primary consideration in magnet quality is the homogeneity or uniformity of the magnetic field. High homogeneity means the magnetic field changes very little over the specified region or volume. The protons in this region resonate at the same frequency in a coherent manner and thus induce the maximum possible signal. One factor affecting magnetic field homogeneity is the magnet design. Large-bore solenoidal magnets generally have the best homogeneity over the largest volume. Short-bore magnets tend to have smaller regions of good homogeneity due to the reduced number of magnet windings used. Open-design magnets will also have reduced regions of good homogeneity. Magnetic field homogeneity is usually expressed in ppm relative to the main field over a certain distance. It is assessed by measuring the field value at various locations inside the magnet and using equation (2.4) to calculate the field variation, replacing the frequencies with the measured magnetic field values. Great effort is taken during magnet manufacturing and installation to ensure the best homogeneity possible. However, manufacturing imperfections or problems with the scan room (e.g., nearby steel posts, asymmetrical metal arrangements) may produce significant field distortions. To analyze and compensate for this, the distortions are characterized by the mathematical shape of the field corrections required as a function of distance away from the magnet center. This classification is referred as the order of the field or shim correction used. First-order or linear corrections in each direction are achieved using the imaging gradient coils described in Section 14.3. Second- or higher-order corrections are nonlinear in nature and most MRI systems use a coil known as a shim coil to correct for them. The design of the shim system may be passive in that it holds pieces of metal (shim plates) or small magnets that correct the field distortions or active in that there are loops of wire through which current passes to correct the field distortions (usually through second order only). In some systems, both types of shim correction may be used. Passive shimming is generally performed at the time of magnet installation as a one-time event. Active shimming (also called electrical shimming) is usually performed on a regular basis during system maintenance and also for each individual patient. Field homogeneity is an important factor to consider when evaluating an MRI system as inadequate homogeneity can cause problems with fat saturation or even general imaging.

14.3 Gradient system

As mentioned in Chapter 4, small linear distortions to $\boldsymbol{B}_0$, known as gradient fields or gradients, are used to localize the tissue signals. Three gradients are used, one each in the x, y, and z directions, to produce the orthogonal field variations required for imaging. They are each generated by the flow of electrical current through separate loops of copper wire mounted into a single form known as the gradient coil. Variations in gradient amplitude are produced by changes in the amount or direction of the current flow through the coil. The current for each gradient axis is provided by an amplifier or power supply. The gradient amplifiers and gradient coils are actively cooled, either by air or chilled water flowing through the components, due to the heat that is generated by the current flow. Gradients are an area where caution should be exercised. Refer to Chapter 16 for a description of safety issues regarding gradients.

One of the major criteria for evaluation of an MRI scanner is the capabilities of the gradient system. There are four aspects that are important in assessing gradient system performance: maximum gradient strength, rise time or slew rate, duty cycle, and techniques for eddy current compensation. Gradient strength is measured in units of mT m^{-1} or G cm^{-1} (1 G cm^{-1} = 10 mT m^{-1}), with typical maximum gradient strengths for current state-of-the-art MRI systems being 40–100 mT m^{-1} (4.0–10.0 G cm^{-1}). These maximum gradient strengths allow thinner slices or smaller FOVs to be obtained without changing other measurement parameters. Another quantity often used to describe maximum gradient amplitudes is the effective gradient amplitude G_{eff} (Figure 14.2). This is the instantaneous vector sum of all three gradients when applied during the scan:

$$G_{eff} = (G_x^2 + G_y^2 + G_z^2)^{1/2} \qquad (14.1)$$

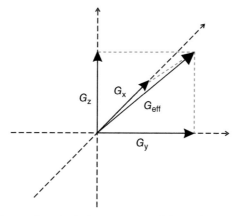

Figure 14.2 The effective gradient G_{eff} is the vector sum of the gradients (G_x, G_y, G_z) in all three directions.

Care must be made to distinguish between the effective gradient and the actual gradient being applied. For example, for a slice selection, orthogonal slices will only use one gradient axis, while only double oblique slices will require all three axes to be active during RF transmission.

The response of a gradient coil to the flow of current is not instantaneous. Gradient pulses require a finite time known as the rise time to achieve their final value. This rise time is nominally 0.1–0.3 ms, which determines a rate of change or slew rate for a gradient pulse. If the desired gradient pulse amplitude is 20 mT m^{-1} with a 0.2 ms rise time, the slew rate is 100 mT m^{-1} ms^{-1} or 100 T m^{-1} s^{-1}. Gradient rise times and/or slew rates are often used to evaluate the performance of the gradient amplifier or power supply producing the current. High-performance amplifiers allow shorter rise times (faster slew rates), enabling shorter gradient pulse durations and/or interpulse delays within a pulse sequence. As a result, the minimum *TE* may be reduced for a given technique while maintaining a small FOV.

The duty cycle of the gradient amplifier is another important measure of gradient performance. The duty cycle determines how long the amplifier can sustain its response to the demands of a pulse sequence. Duty cycles of 100% at the maximum gradient amplitude are typical for state-of-the-art gradient amplifiers for normal imaging sequences. Large duty cycles allow high-amplitude gradient pulses to be used with very short interpulse delays. Low duty cycles mean that the *TE* times will be longer for the scan to allow the gradient amplifiers to return to a standard operating state.

Another complication of gradient pulses is eddy currents. Eddy currents are electric fields produced in a conductive medium by a time-varying magnetic field. In MRI systems, eddy currents are typically induced by the ramping gradient pulse in the body coil located inside the gradient coil and the cryoshield (the innermost portion of the magnet cryostat) outside the coil. These currents generate a magnetic field that opposes and distorts the original gradient pulse. In addition, once the gradient plateau is reached and the ramp is stopped, the eddy currents begin to reduce in amplitude. The net result is that the distorting field will change with time as the eddy currents decay. Therefore the magnetic field homogeneity and the corresponding frequencies change with time as well. Correction of these eddy-current-induced distortions is known as eddy current compensation. Two approaches are commonly used for compensation. One method predistorts the gradient pulse so that the field variation inside the magnet is the desired one. This predistortion may be done via hardware or software. A second approach uses a second set of coil windings surrounding the main gradient coil. This approach is called an actively shielded gradient coil, analogous to the actively shielded magnet described previously. The current flow through the shield coil reduces the eddy currents induced in structures outside the coil. Typical state-of-the-art scanners use both methods of eddy current compensation.

14.4 Radiofrequency system

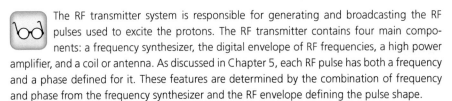 The RF transmitter system is responsible for generating and broadcasting the RF pulses used to excite the protons. The RF transmitter contains four main components: a frequency synthesizer, the digital envelope of RF frequencies, a high power amplifier, and a coil or antenna. As discussed in Chapter 5, each RF pulse has both a frequency and a phase defined for it. These features are determined by the combination of frequency and phase from the frequency synthesizer and the RF envelope defining the pulse shape.

The frequency synthesizer produces the center or carrier frequency for the RF pulse. It also provides the master clock for the measurement hardware during the scan. The frequency synthesizer also provides a phase reference for the scan. Many pulse sequences alternate the phase of the excitation pulse for each line of data by 180° to help reduce stimulated echo artifacts caused by pulse imperfections. Spin echo sequences also typically have the refocusing RF pulses shifted in phase 90° relative to the excitation pulse (known as a Carr–Purcell–Meiboom–Gill, or CPMG, technique). This phase variation may be done through modulation of the RF envelope or of the carrier frequency. More sophisticated synthesizers allow phase changes of 1–2° increments. This finer control also allows for coherence spoiling through incremental phase change of the transmitter, a process known as RF spoiling, used in spoiled gradient echo techniques (Chapter 9).

The RF envelope is generated as a discrete envelope or function containing a range or bandwidth of frequencies. It is made analog and mixed with the carrier frequency prior to amplification to produce an amplitude- or phase-modulated pulse centered at the desired frequency. For some scanners, the final frequency is produced exclusively by the frequency synthesizer, while for other scanners, the RF envelope is modulated to incorporate a frequency offset into the pulse. In either case, the final frequency is determined based on equation (4.1) and generated as a phase coherent signal by the synthesizer.

The RF power amplifier is responsible for producing sufficient power from the frequency synthesizer signal to excite the protons. The amplifier may be solid state or a tube type. In both cases, the amplification is nonlinear in amplitude and phase, causing distortions of the waveform being broadcast. It is necessary to perform some type of nonlinearity correction for the output of the transmitter. Consult the manufacturer for details on the type of correction that is used. Typical RF amplifiers for MR scanners are rated at 2–40 kW of output power at the ^{1}H frequency, with less power required for other nuclei. The actual amount of power required from the amplifier to rotate the protons from equilibrium depends on the field strength, coil transmission efficiency, transmitter pulse duration, and desired excitation angle. This energy deposition in the patient is an area where caution should be exercised. Refer to Chapter 16 on the safety issues regarding the monitoring of RF power deposition.

The final component of the RF system is the transmitter coil. All MR measurements require a transmitter coil or antenna to broadcast the RF pulses. Although transmitter coils can be any size and shape, the one requirement that must be met is that they generate an effective B_1 field perpendicular to B_0. Another feature of most transmitter coils is that they can produce uniform RF excitation over a desired area; that is, a volume can be defined within the coil where all protons experience the same amount of RF energy. Solenoidal MR systems use either a saddle or birdcage coil design, which produces uniform RF excitation even though the coil opening is parallel to B_0. These coils are often adjusted or tuned to the patient to achieve the maximum efficiency in RF transmission. Two types of coil polarity are used: linear polarized (LP) and circularly polarized (CP), also called quadrature. In an LP system, a single coil system is present and the RF pulse is broadcast as a plane wave. A plane wave broadcast at a frequency ω_{TR} has two circularly rotating components, rotating in opposite directions at the same frequency ω_{TR} (Figure 14.3a). For MR, only the component rotating in the same direction as the protons (in-phase) induces resonance absorption. The other component (out-of-phase) is absorbed by the patient as heat. In a CP transmitter system, two coils are present, one rotated 90° from

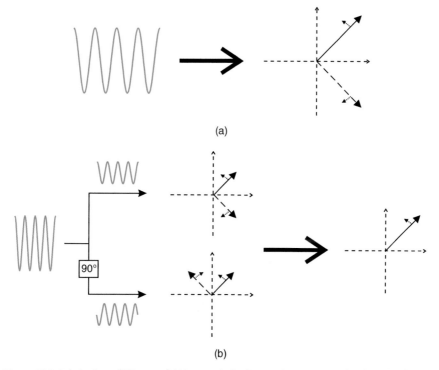

(a)

(b)

Figure 14.3 Polarization of RF wave. (a) Linear polarization. A plane wave can be thought of as the sum of two circular waves rotating in opposite directions. Because the nuclear precession is in only one direction, only one component interacts with the precessing spins (solid arrow) and is effective at resonance absorption. The other component will be absorbed as heat. (b) Circular polarization. A plane wave can be divided into two parts. If one part is shifted 90° relative to the other wave, each part will have one component interacting with the precessing spins (solid arrows), which add together. The counter-rotating components (broken arrows) are always 180° from each other and cancel. The resulting wave is a circular or helical wave with no out-of-phase component.

the other. Phase-shifted RF pulses are broadcast through each coil. The out-of-phase components cancel each other while the in-phase components add coherently (Figure 14.3b). The patient absorbs only the energy from the in-phase components from each coil. A 40% improvement in efficiency from the transmitter system is thereby achieved for a CP system relative to an equivalent LP system for the same proton rotation.

As indicted in Figure 14.3b, the RF waveform broadcast in a CP system is the same waveform except for a phase shift. An alternate approach is to send different waveforms through the two antennas. The waveforms are designed so that the combination provides the desired RF excitation. This concept is referred to as parallel transmission. It has the advantage that a limited volume of tissue can be excited, thereby reducing the SAR. However, multiple transmitter systems are necessary, increasing the cost and complexity of the scanner. Commercial systems implementing parallel transmission have two to four transmitters while ultra-high field systems can have eight or more transmitters.

14.5 Data acquisition system

The data acquisition system is responsible for measuring the signals from the protons and digitizing them for later postprocessing. All MRI systems use a coil to detect the induced voltage from the protons following an RF pulse. The coil is tuned to the particular frequency of the returning signal. This coil may be the same one used to broadcast the RF pulse, or more commonly it may be a dedicated receiver coil. The exact shape and size of the coil are manufacturer-specific, but its effective field must be perpendicular to B_0. The sensitivity of the coil depends on its size, with smaller coils being more sensitive than larger coils but covering a smaller region. Also, the amount of tissue within the sensitive volume of the coil, known as the filling factor, affects the sensitivity. For large-volume studies, such as body or head imaging, the transmitter coil can serve as the receiver coil. For smaller-volume studies, receive-only surface coils are usually used. These coils are small, usually ring-shaped, have high sensitivity but limited penetration, and are used to examine anatomy near the surface of the patient's body. Phased array coils use two or more smaller surface coils to cover a larger area. The small coils are configured so that there is minimal interference between them. This arrangement provides the sensitivity of the small coil but with the anatomical coverage of the larger coil. Current generation scanners have coil arrays containing 4 to 128 individual coils, often referred to as elements.

The signals produced by the protons are usually nV to μV in amplitude and MHz in frequency. In order to process them, amplification is required, which is usually performed in several stages. The initial amplification is performed using a low-noise analog preamplifier located inside the magnet room or built into the coil itself. Further amplification will be performed by the receiver module. Two types of receivers are used in MRI systems. Analog receivers amplify and then demodulate the measured signal relative to the input frequency from the frequency synthesizer to produce a quadrature signal (real and imaginary) with frequencies between 1000 and 250,000 Hz (audio frequency). The signals will be filtered with bandpass filters, then digitized using analog-to-digital converters (ADCs). The ADCs digitize each analog signal at a rate determined by the sampling time and number of data points specified by the user. Typical ADCs can digitize a 10 V signal into 16 bits of information at a rate of 0.1 μs per data point. Digital receivers demodulate the signal to an intermediate frequency and then digitize using an ADC. The final signal amplification, application of a low pass filter, demodulation to an audio range, and quadrature formulation are done on the digital signal. Digital receivers allow for better signal fidelity of the final signal composed to analog receivers. The digitized data are stored on to a hard disk or on to computer memory for later Fourier transformation. Phased array coils typically have a separate preamplifier and ADC for each coil in the array.

Although not formally part of the data acquisition system hardware, an important component of an MRI scanner is RF shielding of the scan room. The weak MR signals must be detected in the presence of background RF signals produced by local radio and television stations. To filter this extraneous noise, MRI scanners are normally enclosed in a copper or stainless steel shield known as a Faraday shield. Maintaining the integrity of this Faraday shield and eliminating in-room sources is very important to minimize noise contamination of the final images.

14.6 Summary of system components

Following is a list of general system features or characteristics to consider in comparing MRI systems, according to subsystem. Individual software features offered by a manufacturer are not included.

Computer systems

Main computer processor speed (GHz)

Capacity of short-term storage disk (Gbytes)

Type of archive device and capacity (Mbytes)

Number and speed of image processors (s image^{-1})

Number of consoles and method of interconnection

Network capability

Filming capabilities

Level and nature of DICOM compliance

Magnet system

Field strength (T)

Field homogeneity measured over a specified diameter of a spherical volume (dsv) (ppm)

0.5 mT (5.0 G) distance from isocenter (in all directions) (m)

Cryogen capacity and evaporation rate (l He day^{-1})

Gradient system

  Maximum gradient amplitude per axis (mT m^{-1} or G cm^{-1})

  Duty cycle (percentage)

  Maximum slew rate (T m^{-1} s^{-1})

  Method(s) of eddy current correction

Radiofrequency system

  RF spoiling capabilities (phase behavior)

  Maximum output power (kW)

  Type of transmitter coils (CP, LP)

  Number of transmitter systems

  Operating frequency range (if multinuclear imaging or spectroscopy is planned)

Data ccquisition system

  Number and type of receiver channels

  Digitization speed of ADCs (minimum μs/point)

  Dynamic range of receiver system, maximum number of available digital bits

  Raw data storage capacity (MGbytes)

  Types of receiver coils (CP, LP, phased array)

  Nature and quality of RF shielding

CHAPTER 15

Contrast agents

One of the strengths of MRI is the significant amount of intrinsic contrast between tissues. This contrast is based upon differences in signal intensity between adjacent pixels representing the tissues in the image. It is a result primarily of differences in the $T1$ and/or $T2$ relaxation times of the tissues under observation accentuated by the chosen TR and TE. In spite of this inherent contrast, it may be challenging to distinguish pathologic from normal tissue. The pathologic tissue may have similar $T1$ or $T2$ times compared to normal tissue. In addition, the voxel may contain significant amounts of normal tissue, which will make the image pixel values similar to those from normal tissue. One approach to increase the signal difference between normal and pathologic tissue is to administer a contrast agent.

Contrast agents for MRI have several advantages over those used for computed tomography (CT). CT agents are direct agents in that they contain an atom (iodine, barium) that attenuates or scatters the incident X-ray beam differently from the surrounding tissue. This scattering permits direct visualization of the agent itself, regardless of its location. Most MRI contrast agents are indirect agents in that they are never visualized directly in the image, but affect the relaxation times of the water protons in the nearby tissue, meaning that one molecule of contrast agent may affect the signal of many nearby spins. The concentration and dosage for MRI agents are therefore significantly lower than for CT agents, which in part explains the lower occurrence of adverse reactions to MRI agents. They are normally excreted through the renal or biliary systems within 24 hours, though the excretion half-time varies substantially from agent to agent. Contrast agents are usually categorized as $T1$ or $T2$ agents based on their primary effect of shortening the $T1$ or $T2$ relaxation times, respectively. However, these agents also shorten the other relaxation times to a lesser degree. The amount of reduction depends on the concentration of the agent: when concentrated, $T1$ agents shorten $T2$ or $T2*$ times and, when dilute, $T2$ agents reduce $T1$ times. Contrast agents may also be grouped into intravenous and oral agents, depending on the route of administration. The following is a brief discussion of MR contrast agents with emphasis on those in current clinical use. Safety issues related to the use of contrast agents are described in Chapter 16.

MRI Basic Principles and Applications, Fifth Edition.
Brian M. Dale, Mark A. Brown and Richard C. Semelka.
© 2015 John Wiley & Sons, Ltd. Published 2015 by John Wiley & Sons, Ltd.

15.1 Intravenous agents

15.1.1 *T1* relaxation agents

Virtually all intravenous contrast agents currently in clinical use are *T1* relaxation agents and are gadolinium-based agents. Gadolinium, a rare earth metal, has a large magnetic moment, but is toxic as a free metallic ion. Gadolinium agents are designed as chelate complexes, which bind to the gadolinium ion and keep it water-soluble, thereby reducing its toxicity. The primary mode of operation for *T1* contrast agents is as a relaxation sink for the water protons.

As mentioned in Chapter 3, *T1* relaxation depends upon the "lattice" receiving the energy that the protons have absorbed from the RF excitation pulse. This energy transfer occurs most efficiently when the protons are in the innermost layer of atoms surrounding the metal ion, known as the coordination sphere. Because the chelate molecules are relatively large and have many bonds to the metal ion, there is limited free space in the inner coordination sphere, which prevents the protons on large molecules such as fat from getting sufficiently close to the metal ion for efficient energy transfer. The tissue water is able to diffuse into the inner coordination sphere of the metal ion and give up its energy, then exchange with the bulk tissue water, enabling additional water molecules to enter the coordination sphere. This diffusion/exchange happens very rapidly ($\sim10^6$ times per second) so that the bulk tissue water is relaxed when the subsequent excitation pulse is applied (Figure 15.1). The result is that the tissue water near the contrast agent has a larger net magnetization M than water in the neighboring tissue and will contribute more signal in a *T1*-weighted image (Figure 15.2). In addition, the rapid exchange process enables many water molecules to be affected by a single chelate complex, which allows low concentrations of contrast agent to be used in clinical studies.

Gadolinium-based contrast agents (GBCAs) are categorized both by the molecular shape of the chelate and by the ionicity of the chelate complex (Figure 15.3). The molecular shape may be linear (the less stable architecture) or macrocyclic, and the ionicity may be nonionic (neutral, less stable) or ionic. Table 15.1 lists the agents that are currently available for clinical use. Many of the agents are nonspecific extracellular agents, in that the agents diffuse rapidly from the vascular space into the interstitial space of the tissue (see Figure 12.4). In the brain, they remain within an intact blood–brain barrier. A relatively small dose (10–20 ml) is typically administered through intravenous injection. The major elimination pathway of these agents is through glomerular filtration and renal excretion. The half-life is typically in the order of 90 minutes with virtually complete elimination of these agents within 24 hours.

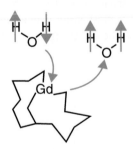

Figure 15.1 Exchange of water molecules in coordination sphere of gadolinium – chelate contrast agent. The chelate molecule causes steric hindrance (crowding) around the gadolinium atom, restricting its access. An excited water molecule is small enough to reach the inner sphere and transfer its energy to the gadolinium ion, then leaves the complex unexcited as another molecule replaces it.

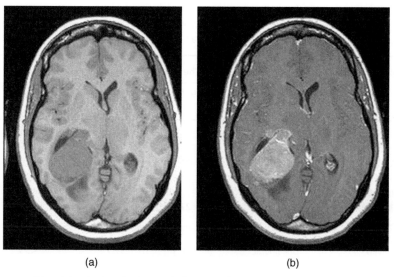

(a)   (b)

Figure 15.2 *T1*-weighted spin echo images before and after administration of gadolinium–chelate contrast agent: (a) no contrast agent present; (b) contrast agent present. Signal increase due to presence of agent.

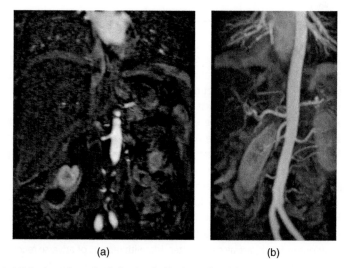

(a)   (b)

Figure 15.3 MRA of renal arteries following half - dose of gadolinium – chelate contrast agent: (a) acquired image from three - dimensional volume acquisition; (b) MIP projection.

Other formulations of gadolinium-chelated contrast agents have both hydrophilic and hydrophobic properties. Two examples of these use benzoxypropionic tetraacetate (BOPTA) and ethoxybenzyl diethylenetriaminepentaacetate (EOB-DTPA) as the ligand. The presence of a hydrophobic ligand enables hepatocyte uptake of these agents and elimination by the biliary system, rather than strictly through renal excretion. Approximately 5% of Gd-BOPTA is eliminated by the hepatobiliary system and 95% by renal excretion, whereas 50% of Gd-EOB-DTPA is eliminated by the hepatobiliary system and 50% by renal excretion. The dual pathways

Table 15.1 Thermodynamic and kinetic stability measurements of gadolinium chelates (from Port et al., 2008). (Abbreviations: K_{cond} = conditional stability constant at physiological pH; K_{therm} = thermodynamic stability constant; $T_{1/2}$ = half-life.)

Gadolinium chelate	Type of structure	Thermodynamic stability		Kinetic stability $T_{1/2}$ at pH 1.0 at 25°C
		log K_{therm}	log K_{cond} (at pH 7.4)	
DOTAREM® (gadoterate meglumine)	Macrocyclic ionic	25.6	19.3	338 h
GADAVIST® (gadobutrol)	Macrocyclic nonionic	21.8	14.7	43 h
PROHANCE® (gadoteridol)	Macrocyclic nonionic	23.8	17.1	3.9 h
MULTIHANCE® (gadobenate dimeglumine)	Linear ionic	22.6	18.4	<5 s
MAGNEVIST® (gadopentate dimeglumine)	Linear ionic	22.1	17.7	<5 s
OMNISCAN™ (gadodiamide)	Linear nonionic	16.9	14.9	<5 s
OPTIMARK™ (gadoversetamide)	Linear nonionic	16.6	15.0	<5 s

of elimination for these agents enable postcontrast imaging emphasizing both tissue perfusion (immediately following administration) and hepatocellular uptake and bile duct elimination (subsequent times). The combined effect of their ease of use and dual-phase behavior have been of significant benefit as liver contrast agents.

The following description of adverse events incorporates information derived from the 2013 Manual on Contrast Media of the American College of Radiology (ACR) (ACR, 2013) and the 2014 Guidelines of the European Society of Urogenital Radiology (ESUR) (Thomsen, 2014).

The frequency of all acute adverse events after an injection of 0.1 or 0.2 mmol kg^{-1} of gadolinium chelate ranges from 0.07% to 2.4%. This frequency is about 8 times higher in patients with a previous reaction to gadolinium-based contrast media. Second reactions can be more severe than the first. Persons with asthma and various other allergies, including allergies to other medications or foods, are also at greater risk, with reports of adverse reaction rates as high as 3.7%. Although there is no cross-reactivity, patients who have had previous allergic-like reactions to iodinated contrast media are also in this category.

Adverse reactions to IV contrast agents can usually be defined as acute, late, and very late events. Acute adverse events occur within 1 hour of contrast medium injection and may manifest as mild, moderate, and severe, with the great majority of reactions being mild. These reactions can be divided into two categories: allergy-like/hypersensitivity and chemotoxic (Table 15.2).

Late adverse events occur 1 h to 1 week after injection and usually manifest as skin reactions similar in type to other drug-induced eruptions (maculopapular rashes, erythema, swelling, and pruritus are most common). This type of reaction has not been described after GBCAs.

Table 15.2   Acute adverse reactions after contrast media injection (from ACR, 2013).

	Allergy-like/hypersensitivity	Chemotoxic
Mild	Mild urticarial	Nausea/mild vomiting
	Mild itching	Warmth/chills
	Erythema	Anxiety
		Vasovagal reaction which resolves spontaneously
Moderate	Marked urticaria	Severe vomiting
	Mild bronchospasm	Vasovagal attack
	Facial/laryngeal edema	
	Vomiting	
Severe	Hypotensive shock	Arrythmia
	Respiratory arrest	Convulsion
	Cardiac arrest	

Very late adverse events usually occur more than 1 week after contrast medium injection and generally reflect deposition of unchelated gadolinium into the extravascular tissues. Unchelated gadolinium is virtually always bound to biologic anions, with phosphates and hydroxyapatites being among the most common biological anions. The most severe recognized form of deposition is termed nephrogenic systemic fibrosis (NSF), which is causally related to the combination of severe acute/chronic renal failure and gadolinium administration. The great majority of NSF cases have occurred in patients in stage 5 chronic renal failure. The classification of chronic renal failure is presented in Table 15.3. The vast majority of cases of NSF are related to the administration of Omniscan, Optimark, or Magnevist, with occurrences of NSF having a frequency of < 1 in 1 million doses in all of the other contrast agents in the setting of their solitary use. Gadolinium is an analog to calcium, and bone deposition in humans has been documented, with a much greater extent of deposition reported to occur with Omniscan compared to Prohance. Currently the long-term consequences from bone deposition have not yet been described. Since children are in a state of much more active bone development it is strongly recommended to only use the most stable gadolinium chelates in pediatric populations. Most recently, a high signal has been described in the basal ganglia of individuals who have undergone multiple repeat MR examinations.

Table 15.3   Chronic kidney disease (CKD) classification based upon the glomerular filtration rate (GFR) (from CKD Work Group, 2013).

GFR stages	GFR (ml/min/1.73 m²)	Terms
G1	>90	Normal or high
G2	60–89	Mildly decreased
G3a	45–59	Mildly to moderately decreased
G3b	30–44	Moderately to severely decreased
G4	15–29	Severely decreased
G5	<15	Kidney failure

15.1.2 *T2* relaxation agents

The other class of intravenous contrast agents are *T2* relaxation agents. They are typically macromolecules containing several iron atoms that collectively form a superparamagnetic center. The large magnetic susceptibility of the macromolecule distorts the local magnetic field in the vicinity of the agent, causing the nearby water protons to dephase more rapidly than the surrounding tissue. This condition results in significant signal loss in *T2*-weighted spin echo or gradient echo images. The most common *T2* contrast agents are based on superparamagnetic iron oxide (SPIO) particulate molecules, also known as ferumoxides. These agents are selectively absorbed by the reticulo-endothelial cells located in the liver, spleen, and bone marrow. Normal tissue in these organ systems take up the agent and have a low signal on *T2*- or *T2**-weighted images. Lesions that do not contain reticulo-endothelial cells in appreciable numbers do not take up the agent and remain unaffected and therefore have a relatively high signal (Figure 15.4).

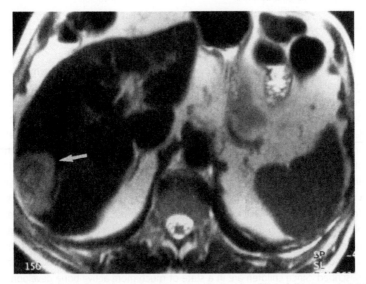

Figure 15.4 *T2*-weighted single-shot echo train spin echo image of liver following administration of superparamagnetic iron oxide contrast agent. The *T2* relaxation times of the normal tissue are reduced by the iron oxide, while the metastatic lesion shows less agent uptake.

Currently, the only *T2* contrast agent licensed for clinical use in the United States is Feridex (magnetite-dextran; Bayer HealthCare AG, Leverkusen, Germany), though its sale was discontinued in the US due to limited sales. It is usually administered as a slow drip infusion over 30 minutes. A further delay of 30 minutes prior to imaging allows for maximal uptake of the agent by reticulo-endothelial cells. Contrast enhancement can be observed from 30 minutes to 4 hours following infusion. Feridex has a good safety profile, but has a potential side effect of acute back pain developing during infusion, occurring in less than 3% of patients. This side effect is usually self-limiting and disappears when the infusion is stopped or slowed. The most important clinical indication for Feridex is in the determination of the extent of liver metastases in patients under consideration for surgical resection. This agent can also distinguish between hepatic origin tumors that contain reticulo-endothelial cells and tumors that do not. Resovist (magnetite/maghemite-carboxydextran; Bayer HealthCare AG, Leverkusen, Germany) is another formulation of a ferumoxide agent that can be administered in a small dose by bolus injection. The advantage of this agent is ease of administration and the lack of back pain as a side effect. It is an ultra-small particulate iron oxide (USPIO) that also increases $T1$ contrast in dynamic gradient echo scanning immediately following administration, enabling one agent to affect both $T1$- and $T2$-weighted scans. Iron-oxide particulate agents are not currently approved for use in liver by the US Food and Drug Administration (FDA).

SPIO agents formulated to a smaller particle size than used for liver imaging are under investigation as contrast agents for the examination of lymph nodes. Normal or hyperplastic lymph nodes take up the agent and lose signal on $T2$-weighted images, whereas malignant lymph nodes do not take up the agent and therefore appear relatively high signal. Iron oxide particles have also been used to label monoclonal antibodies targeted to specific tissue receptor sites. Asioglycan protein receptor contrast agents are one example that is under development.

15.2 Oral agents

Oral MRI contrast agents are typically nonspecific in nature. They are most often used in abdominal and pelvic studies to provide differentiation of bowel from adjacent structures and to provide better delineation of bowel wall processes. Oral agents may be categorized as positive or negative agents. Positive agents increase the overall signal intensity within the image, generally by shortening the $T1$ or $T2$ relaxation times of tissue water. These agents are generally solutions of paramagnetic metal ions or metal–chelate complexes. Many of these agents are present in naturally occurring products (manganese in green tea and blueberry juice) or in over-the-counter medications (ferric ammonium citrate; Geritol; Beecham, Bristol, UK, and Tennessee, US). Other agents have been specifically formulated for use with MRI such as Lumenhance (manganese chloride; Bracco Diagnostic, Princeton, New Jersey, US) and Magnevist Enteral (gadolinium-DTPA; Bayer HealthCare AG, Leverkusen, Germany) as $T1$ relaxation agents and OMR (ferric ammonium citrate; Oncomembrane, Seattle, Washington, US) as a $T2$ relaxation agent. Positive agents can provide excellent delineation of the bowel, but the increased signal may induce greater artifacts as a result of respiratory motion or peristalsis.

The other type of oral contrast agent is a negative agent. Negative agents eliminate the tissue signal from the area of interest. Two approaches are used for negative agents. One method reduces the $T2$ relaxation times using suspensions of ferumoxide particles. The particles may be suspended in aqueous solution (Ferumoxsil; Advanced Magnetics, Cambridge, Massachusetts, US) or adsorbed on to a polymer. The other approach uses an agent that contains no protons and therefore produces no visible MR signal. The most common agent of this type is Perflubron (perfluorooctylbromide (PFOB); Oxygent; Alliance Pharmaceutical, San Diego, California, US). Barium sulfate, clay, and air have also been used for intraluminal studies. One significant problem with many negative contrast agents, particularly iron-based agents and air, is that they increase the local magnetic susceptibility, which may induce significant dephasing artifacts at high field strengths.

For many applications, distention of gastrointestinal segments using water or water-based oral agents may achieve sufficient diagnostic value. For an evaluation of gastric processes, distention with orally administered water may be adequate, while for colorectal processes, endorectal administration of contrast agents is required.

CHAPTER 16

Safety

While considered to be a relatively safe imaging technique, MRI is not without risks. Its use in humans is regulated by healthcare committees of national governments. For example, the US Food and Drug Administration (FDA) has ruled that MRI scanners are Class II medical devices subject to the regulations defined in 21 CFR 892.1000 (US Government, 2008), the same classification as most X-ray-based imaging devices. Operational limits for MRI for most countries are derived from those established by the International Electrotechnical Commission (IEC), with Japan and Italy having separate regulations.

One area where frequent questions arise is pregnancy, both of patients and of workers. While additional research in the area is warranted, there is currently no indication of any adverse biologic effects to the fetus or mother from exposure to the MRI hardware during scanning at any time during the pregnancy (Kanal et al., 2007; Shellock and Crues, 2004). The current recommendations for scanning of pregnant patients is based on the clinical problem under examination and whether MRI is the most appropriate imaging modality to use. Nevertheless, it is prudent to minimize exposure to the MRI scanner during pregnancy, both for patients and health care workers.

There are five general areas where MRI-specific safety precautions are warranted: base magnetic field, cryogens, gradients, RF power deposition, and contrast agents. Depending on the particular scanner and clinical scan in question, one or more of these areas may not be relevant (e.g., a permanent magnet scanner that has no cryogens or a clinical study that does not use contrast media). Manufacturers attempt to minimize any risks through hardware and software limitations on scanning, but some risks cannot be controlled by the manufacturer. Our intention in this section is to describe the potential risks associated with MRI, both for patients and workers, and indicate the current guidelines to minimize these risks.

MRI Basic Principles and Applications, Fifth Edition.
Brian M. Dale, Mark A. Brown and Richard C. Semelka.
© 2015 John Wiley & Sons, Ltd. Published 2015 by John Wiley & Sons, Ltd.

16.1 Base magnetic field

 The first area where precautions should be exercised is the base magnetic field, regardless of its field strength. The examination room in which the magnet is located should have restricted access. Any metal near the magnet should be nonmagnetic (diamagnetic response). Metal items such as stethoscopes or pens may be attracted to the magnet, causing possible injury. Breathing gases used for sedated patients should be either built into the wall or supplied from nonferrous tanks. Electrical equipment must be protected or shielded from the magnetic field in order to function properly. Patients with surgical implants or metal fragments in their bodies as a result of trauma or occupation (e.g., sheet metal workers) should be scanned only if there is no risk to the patient should the implant or fragment move during the procedure. Patients with magnetic pacemakers, or ferromagnetic intracranial aneurysm clips, or neurostimulators should not be scanned under any circumstances due to the risk of patient injury. The magnetic properties of various medical implants have been extensively described by Shellock and coworkers (Shellock and Spinazzi, 2008).

It is also important to realize that the magnetic field of all magnets extends in all directions away from the center of the field, including vertically. The amount of fringe magnetic field (the portion outside the magnet housing) is a very important consideration in siting an MRI system. The fringe field is greatest near the magnet parallel to the field (typically in the z direction) and decreases with increasing distance away from the magnet. The fringe field is also larger for higher field magnets. A low-field magnet has a very small fringe field, making it easier to use standard patient monitoring equipment. High-field systems are often manufactured with magnetic shielding of different types to reduce the fringe field. This shielding may surround the magnet (passive shielding), be generated by a second set of superconducting magnet windings surrounding the main field (active shielding), or be built into the wall (room shielding). Two distances are of concern regarding the fringe field. The 0.5 mT (5 G) distance is considered the minimum safe distance for persons with conventional pacemakers. This distance prevents interference of the pacemaker operation by the magnetic field. An important study describes MRI-compatible pacemakers (Sommer et al., 2006; Nazarian et al., 2006) that have been developed and are in clinical use in Europe. The 0.1 mT (1 G) distance, the nominal distance for other equipment that uses cathode ray tube monitors, prevents distortion of the image on the monitor by the magnetic field. The actual distances are installation- and equipment-specific. Contact the manufacturer regarding individual situations.

16.2 Cryogens

Most MRI magnets are manufactured with wire that becomes superconducting when immersed in liquid helium, an example of a cryogen. Cryogens are very cold liquids, specifically helium or nitrogen, which are used in superconducting magnets to maintain the magnetic field. These liquids boil at temperatures well below 0 °C (helium at −270 °C, nitrogen at −196 °C). During refilling of the magnets with these liquids, contact with the transfer line can cause frostbite. In addition, the occurrence of a quench or spontaneous discharge of the magnet will cause the energy within the magnet windings to heat up the interior of the magnet. This heat will cause the helium liquid to boil, increasing its volume by three orders of magnitude. Manufacturers connect exhaust pipes to vent this gas to the exterior of the building so that the gas will escape harmlessly. However, should this vent become occluded, the gas will escape into the scan room, displacing the oxygen. In the event of a quench, all personnel and patients should evacuate the scan room.

16.3 Gradients

One area of concern with gradients is the potential for the stimulation of nerve tissue produced by the change in B_0 caused by the gradient. If the change in B_0 is large and rapid enough (represented by the quantity dB/dt), then nerve stimulation may occur. The greatest area for this is at the edge of the gradient coil, as this is where the gradient amplitude change is greatest. This corresponds to the entrance to the bore for a solenoidal magnet. Manufacturers are required by the governing regulatory organizations (FDA, IEC, etc.) to limit dB/dt so that no cardiac stimulation occurs due to the gradient pulsing. Because of the directional nature of the gradients and the nerve tissue, scan protocols may be limited in one direction more than another to reduce the potential for stimulation. Limitations in a scan protocol are most frequently encountered when rapid gradient pulsing is used, such as in echo planar sequences, or gradient echo sequences with a small FOV and short TR, as in cardiovascular imaging.

A second area of concern with gradients is acoustic noise. The gradients are generated by electrical currents and a mechanical force is produced in the gradient coil winding as a result of interactions with the base magnetic field. This process is the same as used in a loudspeaker connected to an audio amplifier. The amount of noise generated in an MR scan depends on the rate and strength of gradient pulsing. Different pulse sequences will create different amounts of acoustic noise (e.g., spin echo versus echo planar imaging). Also, certain operator parameters will affect the volume; for example, small FOV, thin slices, short TR. In many cases, hearing protection for the patient may be advised.

16.4 RF power deposition

Although MR is considered a relatively safe imaging technique, the $T1$ relaxation process converts the absorbed RF power to heat inside the patient. Manufacturers are required by the governing regulatory organizations (FDA, IEC, etc.) to have two monitors, either hardware or software, to limit the RF power deposited in a patient (IEC). This is to ensure that excessive patient heating does not occur over both the excited tissue volume (localized) and the entire patient (whole body). To accomplish this, the specific absorption rate of energy dissipation or SAR is monitored. The SAR is measured in watts of energy per kilogram of patient body weight (W kg^{-1}). MRI systems are designed to operate at or below the SAR guidelines, which are set to limit the core body temperature rise to approximately 1 °C or less, with slightly higher elevations allowed for regional examinations. For low-field scanners, the SAR seldom limits the measurement protocols. For high-field scanners, the SAR limits have a significant effect on the number of slices or saturation pulses that can be applied to the patient within a scan. The major challenge is in the estimation of the amount of tissue exposed to the RF energy. This depends on the nature and transmission profile of the transmitter coil as well as the patient size. Consult the manufacturer for specific details on the SAR monitoring system that is incorporated into a particular scanner.

16.5 Contrast media

 In general, MR contrast agents have a relatively good safety record. Adverse reactions to the presence of the media have been rare. However, there have been reports of nephrogenic systemic fibrosis (NSF) occurring in patients with acute or class 4 or 5 chronic renal failure when administered gadolinium-based contrast agents (Kuo et al., 2007). While not present in all cases, most of the patients who developed NSF were given high dosages (frequently used for angiographic studies) of nonionic agents. The hypothesis is that the stability of these compounds, both kinetic and thermodynamic, is less than for the ionic linear and macrocyclic agents. As a result, unchelated gadolinium is present in larger concentrations, leading to increased deposition in tissues, primarily the skin. The US FDA issued a "black box" warning (US Food and Drug Administration, 2006) recommending against the use of gadolinium-based contrast media for patients with renal insufficiency unless the diagnostic information is essential and cannot be obtained using a noncontrast technique.

A second group of patients for which contrast media is not recommended is pregnant patients. While there are no studies to suggest that there is a risk to the fetus by contrast media, caution should be used in performing these studies. Bone deposition is a potentially serious complication of gadolinium contrast use in the fetus and children, as gadolinium is a calcium analog and can be taken up in bone. Nonionic linear agents should not be used for these patients.

CHAPTER 17

Clinical applications

In selecting pulse sequences and measurement parameters for a specific application, MRI allows the user tremendous flexibility to produce variations in contrast between normal and diseased tissue. This flexibility is available when imaging both stationary tissue as well as flowing blood. For example, the use of both bright blood and dark blood MRA techniques described in Chapter 12 permits more accurate assessment of vascular patency and intravascular mass lesions. A typical patient examination acquires multiple series of images with different types of contrast (proton density, $T1$, $T2$) and different slice orientations (transverse, sagittal, coronal, oblique), providing the clinician with more complete information on the nature of the tissue under observation and increasing the likelihood of lesion detection and correct characterization. It is critical that the scan protocols be appropriate for the disease process under investigation, the organ or organs being imaged, and the individual patient. For example, breath-hold scans may not be possible for some patients. Also, an incorrect choice of scan parameters may render the diseased tissue to be isointense with the normal tissue. The MR physician may choose to provide detailed measurement parameters for each examination or have a predetermined regimen of scans that are to be performed by a technologist. Establishing fixed measurement protocols ensures the efficient operation of the MR scanner and that reliable, reproducible imaging examinations are performed. We advocate the second approach for clinical scanning.

17.1 General principles of clinical MR imaging

There are three fundamental principles that should guide the development of MRI scan protocols:
1 Accurate and reproducible image quality.
2 Good visualization of disease processes.
3 Comprehensive imaging information for the area under observation.

MRI Basic Principles and Applications, Fifth Edition.
Brian M. Dale, Mark A. Brown and Richard C. Semelka.
© 2015 John Wiley & Sons, Ltd. Published 2015 by John Wiley & Sons, Ltd.

Because ideal achievement of all three goals may not be practical, pulse sequences and/or scan parameters should be chosen that will provide adequate results within a clinically acceptable scan time. However, careful consideration should be made in prescribing scan protocols as the ability to visualize disease relative to normal tissue can be dramatically affected by improper scan protocols. One common approach to enhance the contrast between abnormal and background tissue is to make the signal of one of the tissues significantly different from the other one. For example, variation of the signal of fat through the use of unsuppressed and fat-suppressed techniques aids in the detection of lymph nodes. On *T1*-weighted images, lymph nodes have a low signal and therefore are conspicuous in a background of high signal fat, while on *T2*-weighted images, lymph nodes are relatively bright and their conspicuity is improved by decreasing the signal of background fat using fat suppression techniques. Following administration of a gadolinium-chelated contrast agent, lymph nodes have significantly shorter *T1* values and produce a moderately high signal on *T1*-weighted images. The use of fat suppression is helpful to reduce the competing high signal of fat. The combined use of gadolinium-chelated contrast agents and fat suppression to increase the signal of diseased tissue and to decrease the signal from background fat, respectively, is widely used in various organ systems including the orbits, the bony skeleton, soft tissue of the extremities, and the breast.

An additional consideration is in the choice of pulse sequence, in that there may be differences in signal from flowing tissue or dramatic differences in image quality. For example, fat-suppressed spoiled gradient echo may be preferable to fat-suppressed spin echo when a concomitant evaluation of patency of vessels is desired, as in assessing vascular grafts for patency or infection, or for imaging extremities to determine soft tissue infection or vascular thrombosis. This is because spoiled gradient echo images display high signal intensity for patent vessels and low signal intensity for occluded vessels when acquired within a time window of 2–5 minutes following administration of gadolinium-chelated contrast media. In comparison, spin echo images may have a signal void from both patent and thrombosed vessels. Flowing tissue is commonly seen as a signal void on spin echo images due to the dephasing of moving spins during the gradient pulses, while blood clots produce a low signal due to the presence of fibrinous clot and increased *T2** effects from blood breakdown products.

It is important when defining protocols for MRI studies to obtain a sufficient variety of sequences to provide comprehensive information, while at the same time not to be too redundant and generate excessively long exams. For example, our approach for imaging of the abdomen has been to employ a variety of short-duration *T1*- and *T2*-weighted sequences with the majority of them performed in the transverse plane, but also obtain at least one set of images in a plane orthogonal to the transverse plane. The particular choice of image orientation and number of slices for a measurement is dictated by the area of anatomy under observation.

17.2 Examination design considerations

The initial studies of MRI used primarily transverse $T1$- and $T2$-weighted spin echo techniques. As the modality has matured, it has become clear that imaging strategies must be modified beyond this elementary approach. There are several reasons for this:

1 Imaging of organs in the plane of the best anatomical display. Imaging of the spine or the female pelvis requires the use of both sagittal and transverse images to best demonstrate the anatomical structures. Similarly, the evaluation of large masses in the region of the upper poles of the kidneys is facilitated by sagittal as well as transverse images. On the other hand, coronal images are useful for visualization of the left lobe of the liver. Some organs, such as cardiac MRI, have organ-specific planes that are particularly useful but are oblique to the standard planes mentioned above.

2 Compensation for the most severe artifacts generated by various organ systems. Abdominal imaging is severely compromised by artifacts from respiratory motion. Imaging protocols that employ breath-hold spoiled gradient echo sequences (e.g., FLASH, spoiled GRASS), as described in Chapter 10, can produce images with substantial $T1$-weighting while minimizing respiratory artifacts. Cardiac gating is useful when imaging the thorax in order to minimize phase artifacts from cardiac motion. Three-dimensional volume gradient echo techniques are superior to 2D techniques for $T1$-weighted imaging of lungs, because the 3D techniques exhibit fewer phase artifacts from flowing blood and cardiac motion.

3 Increased spatial resolution and/or signal-to-noise. Imaging of small anatomical regions such as extremities (e.g., ankles, wrists, knees) or the breast require specialized surface coils to maximize both signal-to-noise and spatial resolution.

4 The use of contrast agents. Imaging of nonorgan-deforming focal lesions in the liver, spleen, and pancreas using intravenous gadolinium-based contrast agents requires rapid, breath-hold imaging techniques to capture the capillary phase of lesion enhancement. This approach necessitates the use of spoiled gradient echo techniques (e.g., FLASH or spoiled GRASS, either 2D or 3D versions) with temporal resolution of less than 20 seconds. In many instances, the visualization of contrast enhancement in $T1$-weighted images may be improved through the use of fat suppression to remove the competing high signals from fat.

17.3 Protocol considerations for anatomical regions

The following considerations and recommendations are offered for imaging various organ systems. They are intended to indicate general guidelines for use in developing imaging examinations. Exact sequence protocols are not provided because different manufacturers have different imaging capabilities and functions.

17.3.1 Brain

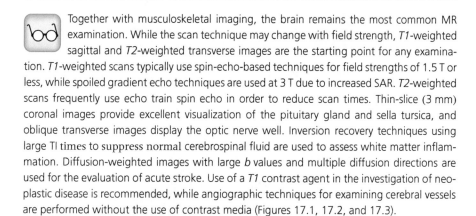

Together with musculoskeletal imaging, the brain remains the most common MR examination. While the scan technique may change with field strength, *T1*-weighted sagittal and *T2*-weighted transverse images are the starting point for any examination. *T1*-weighted scans typically use spin-echo-based techniques for field strengths of 1.5 T or less, while spoiled gradient echo techniques are used at 3 T due to increased SAR. *T2*-weighted scans frequently use echo train spin echo in order to reduce scan times. Thin-slice (3 mm) coronal images provide excellent visualization of the pituitary gland and sella tursica, and oblique transverse images display the optic nerve well. Inversion recovery techniques using large TI times to suppress normal cerebrospinal fluid are used to assess white matter inflammation. Diffusion-weighted images with large *b* values and multiple diffusion directions are used for the evaluation of acute stroke. Use of a *T1* contrast agent in the investigation of neoplastic disease is recommended, while angiographic techniques for examining cerebral vessels are performed without the use of contrast media (Figures 17.1, 17.2, and 17.3).

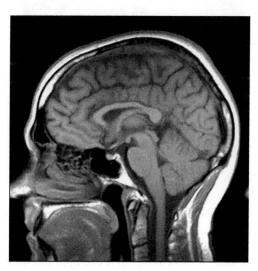

Figure 17.1 Sagittal spin echo *T1*-weighted head image. *TR*, 500 ms; *TE*, 7.7 ms.

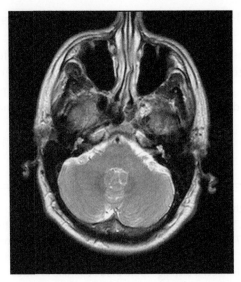

Figure 17.2 Transverse echo train spin echo *T2*-weighted head image. *TR*, 4000 ms; effective *TE*, 100 ms; echo train length, 5.

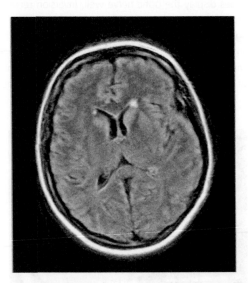

Figure 17.3 Transverse echo train spin echo fluid attenuated head image, *TR*, 9000 ms; effective *TE*, 87 ms; *TI*, 2500 ms.

17.3.2 Neck

The use of a surface coil for neck imaging is essential due to the small volume of tissue under examination. High resolution *T1*- and *T2*-weighted sequences are useful for visualizing soft tissue. The use of gadolinium-based contrast agents may be helpful for tumor and lymph node detection, and for thyroid and parathyroid studies. The addition of fat suppression to postcontrast studies is helpful to delineate tissue. Uniform fat suppression may be difficult to achieve due to magnetic field distortions from the large magnetic susceptibility differences between the neck and the upper thorax.

17.3.3 Spine

A combination of *T1*- and *T2*-weighted images is important. Both sagittal and transverse images are valuable for examining the spinal cord and structural deformations such as disk herniations (Figures 17.4, 17.5, and 17.6). Transverse

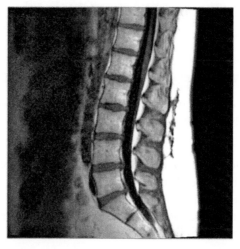

Figure 17.4 Sagittal echo train spin echo *T1*-weighted lumbar spine image. *TR*, 550 ms; effective *TE*, 11 ms; echo train length, 3. Anterior spatial presaturation pulse is used to suppress peristalsis and respiration artifacts.

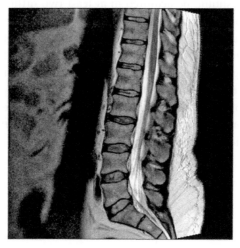

Figure 17.5 Sagittal echo train *T2*-weighted lumbar spine image. *TR*, 4000 ms; effective *TE*, 87 ms; echo train length, 17. Anterior spatial presaturation pulse is used to suppress peristalsis and respiration artifacts.

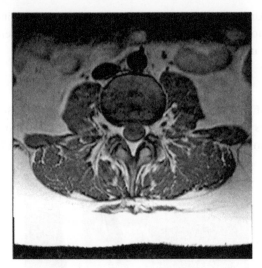

Figure 17.6 Transverse echo train spin echo *T1*-weighted lumbar spine image. *TR*, 764 ms; effective *TE*, 11 ms; echo train length, 3.

images allow excellent visualization of nerve roots and possible disk fragments. Use of spatial presaturation pulses is recommended to reduce artifacts from jaw, tongue, or esophageal motion in cervical studies or abdominal motion in lumbar studies. Administration of gadolinium-based contrast media and fat suppression are recommended in circumstances in which bony metastases are suspected.

17.3.4 Musculoskeletal

A combination of *T1*- and *T2*-weighted images is routinely used in musculoskeletal imaging. Images should be acquired in at least two orthogonal planes with high spatial resolution to ensure proper anatomical visualization (Figures 17.7, 17.8, and 17.9). Fat suppressed images are frequently valuable for detection of tumor, inflammation, or avascular necrosis and may replace *T2*-weighted images in some settings (Figure 17.10). *T2**-weighted images are often used for visualizing fluid and bony detail. Use of gadolinium-based contrast agents is important for the evaluation of inflammatory and neoplastic disease, often in combination with fat suppression. When imaging small anatomical regions away from the magnet isocenter, field homogeneity may limit the usefulness of fat suppression (Figures 17.11 and 17.12).

17.3.5 Thorax

Cardiac triggering may be of value to minimize motion artifacts from the heart. Transverse *T1*-weighted images provide good anatomical evaluation of the mediastinum and chest wall. *T2*-weighted transverse images are helpful, particularly in the evaluation of chest wall or mediastinal involvement with cancer.

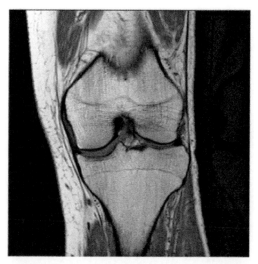

Figure 17.7 Coronal spin echo *T1*-weighted knee image. *TR*, 570 ms; *TE*, 12 ms.

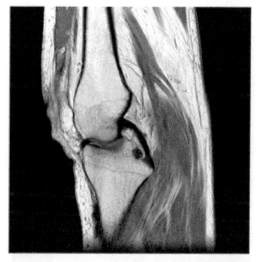

Figure 17.8 Sagittal echo train spin echo proton density–weighted knee image. *TR*, 3000 ms; effective *TE*, 27 ms; echo train length, 6.

T1-weighted images acquired following administration of gadolinium-based contrast media provide similar and complementary information. Fat suppression is a useful adjunct when gadolinium-based contrast agents are employed. The lowered signal from fat improves the visualization of abnormal tissue enhancement, which is helpful for delineating the presence of chest wall invasion by malignant or infectious processes. Lesions in the lung apex and occasionally in the lung base require additional coronal or sagittal views. Breath-hold imaging following administration of gadolinium-based contrast media improves

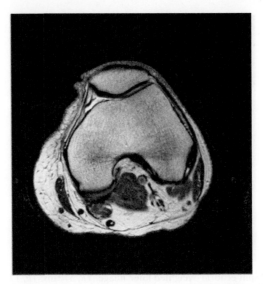

Figure 17.9 Transverse echo train spin echo proton density–weighted knee image. *TR*, 4100 ms; effective *TE*, 27 ms; echo train length, 11.

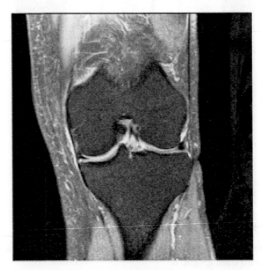

Figure 17.10 Coronal echo train spin echo proton density–weighted knee image with fat saturation. *TR*, 3000 ms; effective *TE*, 26 ms; echo train length, 6.

visualization of small peripheral lung lesions; metastases can be reliably seen at a diameter of 5 mm at 1.5 T and at 3.5 mm at 3.0 T using this approach. A 3D gradient echo sequence is preferred for imaging lung parenchyma because the technique minimizes phase artifacts from cardiac motion. For most examinations, imaging between 2 and 5 minutes following contrast administration provides a good balance between contrast enhancement of lung masses with

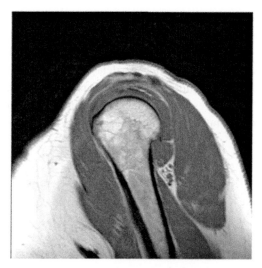

Figure 17.11 Oblique sagittal spin echo *T1*-weighted shoulder image. *TR*, 433 ms; *TE*, 10 ms.

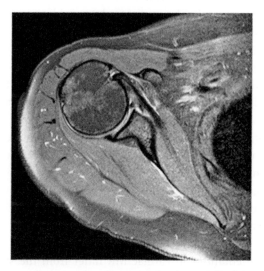

Figure 17.12 Transverse echo train spin echo proton density–weighted shoulder image with fat saturation. *TR*, 3000 ms; effective *TE*, 37 ms; echo train length, 7.

diminished enhancement of the blood pool. The prolonged retention of contrast in the vascular space in MR, compared to CT using iodinated contrast media, is advantageous for visualization of patent pulmonary arteries.

17.3.6 Breast

Optimal breast MR examination requires a dedicated multichannel breast coil to maximize spatial resolution. *T1*-weighted imaging using thin-slice 3D volume techniques are routinely used incorporating fat suppression. Lesion detection is achieved using serial, dynamic imaging following gadolinium-based contrast media administration and provides useful information on lesion characterization (see Figure 12.5). Many carcinomas exhibit intense early enhancement while most benign disease processes enhance in a delayed, less intense fashion. Further information regarding lesion morphology may be provided using high-resolution *T2*-weighted ETSE sequences. Morphology of lesions on gadolinium-enhanced *T1*-weighted images has become the primary method for lesion evaluation.

17.3.7 Heart and great vessels

Transverse cardiac-triggered *T1*-weighted segmented gradient echo sequences are essential in the evaluation of cardiac anatomy. When possible, breath-hold scanning, real-time imaging, or use of navigator echoes is preferred to minimize artifacts from respiratory motion. High spatial resolution is frequently needed, particularly in assessing congenital heart disease; therefore, a slice thickness of less than 5 mm is recommended. Coronal and sagittal triggered *T1*-weighted images may provide additional information in many instances. They are essential in the evaluation of congenital heart disease by providing anatomical information regarding vessels, airways, and cardiac chambers. The left anterior oblique sagittal plane is an important view for the evaluation of the thoracic aorta.

The signal from flowing blood within the cardiac chambers is often heterogeneous as a result of changes in flow direction and velocity. For *T1*-weighted sequences, it is helpful to minimize the blood signal, both to reduce flow artifacts and to delineate vessels using dark blood techniques (Figure 17.10). Application of superior and inferior presaturation pulses or gradient dephasing may be required. Flow compensation should be avoided because it results in an increased signal from flowing blood. Alternately, refocused gradient echo techniques that produce a high signal from flowing blood (bright blood techniques) are used for the evaluation of chamber dynamics. Multiphasic techniques (cine MR) are particularly useful in the evaluation of wall motion and thickening, valvular disease, and shunts.

Useful image orientations in cardiac MR differ from the standard imaging planes used elsewhere and are tailored to the cardiac anatomy, which is usually in a double-oblique orientation with respect to the standard planes and varies from person to person. The short-axis view is useful for evaluating the pulmonary valve and for performing volumetric measurements (Figure 17.13). The four-chamber view is useful for evaluating septal defects, chamber size, the lateral walls and apex of the left ventricle, and the free wall of the right ventricle (Figure 17.14). Other views can be tailored to examine the major vessels and valves (Figure 17.15), the coronary vessels, or the left ventricle long axis. Single-shot echo train spin echo techniques can minimize cardiac motion artifacts and are useful as bright or dark blood techniques. For the evaluation of the aorta and major branches, a widely used technique is MR angiography

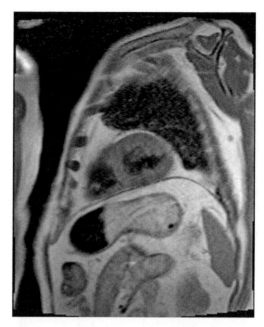

Figure 17.13 Short axis echo train spin echo dark-blood cardiac image. *TR*, 1142 ms; effective *TE*, 32 ms; echo train length, 21.

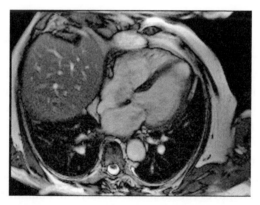

Figure 17.14 Four-chamber steady-state gradient echo bright-blood cardiac image. *TR*, 36.1 ms; *TE*, 1.8 ms.

employing a dynamic 3D gradient echo sequence following gadolinium-based contrast media administration.

17.3.8 Liver

Both *T1*- and *T2*-weighted transverse images are important for evaluating the liver. Combining breath-hold and nonbreath-hold sequences is often useful since

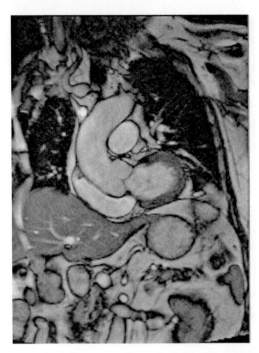

Figure 17.15 Oblique coronal steady-state gradient echo bright-blood heart image. *TR*, 35.5 ms; *TE*, 1.8 ms.

some patients can suspend respiration but cannot breathe regularly, while other patients breathe regularly but cannot hold their breath well. Most current protocols combine breath-hold *T1*- and *T2*-weighted sequences with breathing independent *T2*-weighted sequences. A spoiled gradient echo sequence is most often used for *T1*-weighted imaging, either 2D or 3D, assuming that very short *TE* are used; however, *T1*-weighted spin echo with respiratory compensation may be considered for some patients. When the image quality is acceptable, 3D techniques are preferred. For *T2*-weighted images, breathing averaged ETSE with fat suppression is a useful technique. The addition of fat suppression diminishes respiratory ghosts, removes chemical shift artifacts, and diminishes the signal of a fatty infiltrated liver, which permits good visualization of the liver capsular surface and facilitates lesion detection. In many cases, *T2*-weighted single-shot ETSE techniques acquired with and without fat suppression may be sufficient (Figures 17.16–17.18, and 17.19).

The use of intravenous contrast agents significantly improves lesion detection over nonenhanced imaging techniques. Currently available contrast agents include various gadolinium-based complexes for *T1* enhancement and ferumoxides for *T2* enhancement. When using gadolinium-based contrast agents, it is important to image early after contrast (~30 seconds) to maximize the specific enhancement features of various focal hepatic lesions (Figure 17.19). Spoiled

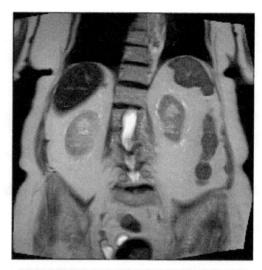

Figure 17.16 Coronal single-shot echo train *T2*-weighted image of liver and kidneys. Effective *TE*, 94 ms.

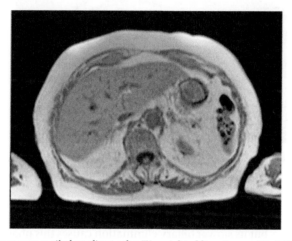

Figure 17.17 Transverse spoiled gradient echo *T1*-weighted liver image. *TR*, 182 ms; *TE*, 4.4 ms; excitation angle, 70°.

gradient echo techniques (2D or 3D) are extremely useful to accomplish this goal. In addition, serial sequence repetition with additional acquisitions at approximately 1 and 2 minutes postcontrast may be routinely useful to visualize the temporal behavior of contrast uptake.

While contrast agents are used primarily to assess early perfusion of the liver, there are agents that also provide good contrast for hepatocyte phase imaging. Eovist is a gadolinium-chelate agent with hepatocyte phase imaging available 20 minutes following injection, facilitating both early perfusion and late hepatocyte phase imaging in one 20 minute study. Multihance also possesses a

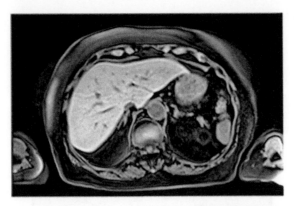

Figure 17.18 Transverse three-dimensional volume *T1*-weighted spoiled gradient echo liver image with fat suppression. *TR*, 4.9 ms; *TE*, 2.4 ms; excitation angle, 10°.

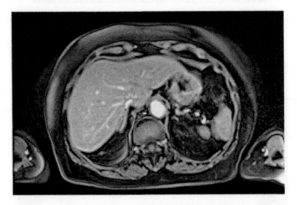

Figure 17.19 Transverse three-dimensional volume spoiled gradient echo *T1*-weighted liver image with fat suppression, following gadolinium – chelate contrast administration. *TR*, 4.9 ms; *TE*, 2.4 ms; excitation angle, 10°.

hepatocyte phase, but its slower biliary elimination causes this phase to occur one hour following contrast administration, requiring careful time management of the scanner and patient. Currently, the advantages of Eovist include the shorter hepatocyte phase development time and better visualization of the biliary tree compared to Multihance. Significant disadvantages include increased cost and lesser hepatic arterial enhancement when using approved dosages.

While not yet established as routine practice at all centers, the use of diffusion-weighted imaging is drawing increasing attention for hepatic applications. The motion sensitivity of diffusion poses challenges in the abdomen, as does the off-resonance sensitivity of the EPI readout. As a result, both shimming and respiratory techniques are important, with some centers using a breath-hold approach, others using a free-breathing approach, and still others using a respiratory navigator approach. All three approaches have drawbacks and limitations that can render them undiagnostic, but, when successful, abdominal DWI generates a high image contrast between normal liver parenchyma and malignant lesions.

17.3.9 Abdominal organs

T1-weighted breath-hold spoiled gradient echo techniques, either 2D or 3D, are useful for controlling respiratory artifacts in the abdomen. When the image quality is acceptable, 3D techniques are preferred. As with the liver, combining breath-hold with breathing independent sequences are advantageous. Single-shot ETSE *T2*-weighted sequences are particularly effective at demonstrating bowel and for distinguishing bowel from other entities. Transverse fat-suppressed and conventional spoiled gradient echo images are useful in combination both prior to and following administration of intravenous gadolinium-based contrast agents. Following contrast administration, the unsuppressed technique is useful to visualize capillary phase enhancement, while the subsequent acquisition of the fat-suppressed technique provides interstitial phase information. For the kidneys and pancreas, dynamic acquisition of fat-suppressed 3D gradient echo images enables excellent organ visualization. Imaging of the adrenal glands require noncontrast out-of-phase gradient echo images (Figures 17.20, 17.21, and 17.22).

17.3.10 Pelvis

Transverse images are routinely used, while sagittal images provide a useful adjunct. *T1*-weighted images are frequently best performed as conventional spin echo or spoiled gradient echo (either 2D or 3D), whereas *T2*-weighted

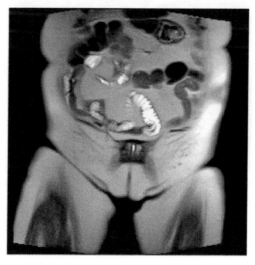

Figure 17.20 Coronal single-shot echo train *T2*-weighted image of bowel. Effective *TE*, 94 ms.

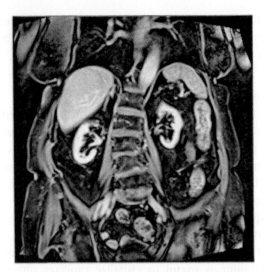

Figure 17.21 Coronal three-dimensional volume spoiled gradient echo *T1*-weighted image of kidneys with fat suppression, following gadolinium – chelate contrast administration. *TR*, 4.9 ms; *TE*, 2.4 ms; excitation angle, 10°.

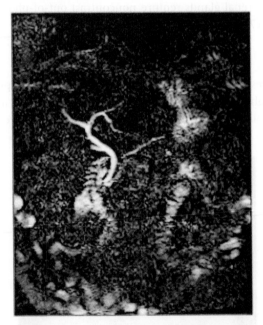

Figure 17.22 Coronal single-shot echo train spin echo *T2*-weighted image of common bile duct, following fat suppression. *TR*, 3450 ms; effective *TE*, 1200 ms; *TI*, 150 ms.

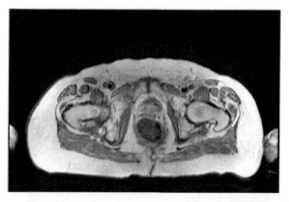

Figure 17.23 Transverse echo train spin echo proton density–weighted image of pelvis. *TR,* 4500 ms; effective *TE*, 20 ms; echo train length, 7.

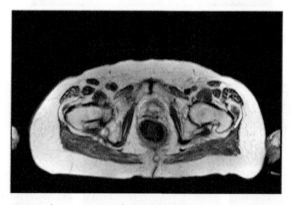

Figure 17.24 Transverse echo train spin echo proton density–weighted image of pelvis. *TR,* 4500 ms; effective *TE*, 101 ms; echo train length, 7.

images may be acquired as breathing-averaged ETSE or single-shot ETSE. Thin slices (5 mm thickness) in the sagittal plane are necessary to optimally visualize the uterus and ovaries in the female and the seminal vesicles in the male (Figures 17.23, 17.24, and 17.25). Detailed imaging of the pelvis also requires high in-plane spatial resolution (512 × 512 matrices, ETSE, small FOV). *T2*-weghted scans, acquired as thin-slice 3D acquisitions, are useful for mulitplanar reconstruction. Gadolinium-based contrast administration is important in the evaluation of uterine and adnexal masses as well as in the evaluation and characterization of other pelvic masses such as rectal tumors. Fat suppression is an important adjunct to contrast administration when ovarian cancer is clinically suspected. Diffusion-weighted imaging is gaining acceptance for management of prostate cancer (Figure 17.26).

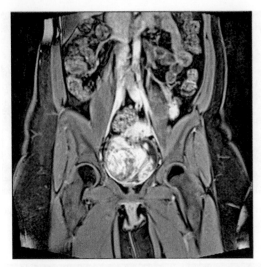

Figure 17.25 Coronal three-dimensional volume spoiled gradient echo image, following gadolinium–chelate contrast administration. *TR*, 4.9 ms; *TE*, 2.4 ms; excitation angle, 10°.

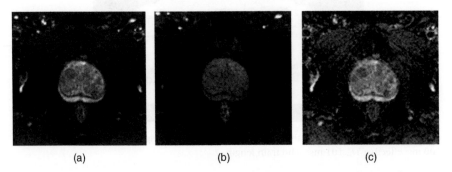

(a)   (b)   (c)

Figure 17.26 Diffusion-weighted imaging of the prostate at 3 T: (a) *b*-value, 50 s mm^{-2}; (b) *b*-value, 800 s mm^{-2}; (c) apparent diffusion coefficient map. Courtesy of Siemens AG, in cooperation with Dr. Engelhardt, Hospital Martha-Maria, Nuernberg, Germany.

17.4 Recommendations for specific sequences and clinical situations

17.4.1 *T1*-weighted techniques
Single echo spin echo
For routine *T1*-weighted imaging, a moderate *TR* is recommended (400–700 ms at 1.0 and 1.5 T) with a short *TE* (20 ms or less). This combination allows acquisition of a sufficient number of slices yet provides acceptable contrast between most tissues. The slice thickness and in-plane spatial resolution can be tailored

to the particular anatomical region under examination. Spin echo sequences are typically not used at 3 T due to increased limitations from SAR.

Spoiled gradient echo

Imaging parameters include a relatively long TR (~140 ms) and the shortest in-phase echo time (4.5 ms at 1.5 T, 2.25 ms at 3.0 T) for unsuppressed or an opposed-phase echo time for fat suppressed imaging, one signal average, and an excitation angle of 70–90°. These parameters maximize the number of slices, SNR, and $T1$-weighting, yet minimize artifacts and the measurement time. This spoiled gradient echo sequence is ideal for $T1$-weighted imaging in the abdomen, for imaging in multiple planes, and for imaging following administration of intravenous gadolinium-based contrast media. It is also a standard method for obtaining $T1$-weighted images at 3 T or higher. In general, 3D techniques are preferred over 2D techniques on current generation MR scanners, as the complete imaging volume can be scanned and thinner slices can be obtained. These require a minimal TR and a reduced flip angle. The use of parallel imaging techniques allows an image of high spatial resolution to be acquired.

Out-of-phase gradient echo

Imaging parameters should include the shortest possible opposed-phase TE (1.1 ms at 3.0 T, 2.25 ms at 1.5 T), which must be shorter than the in-phase TE used. This technique allows easy detection of fat and water in similar proportions within a tissue volume through signal cancellation. For clinical use, the most important applications for this technique are the examination for fatty infiltration of liver and for benign adrenal adenoma. In both cases, the observation of signal drop observed on out-of-phase images compared to in-phase images permits the diagnosis of fatty infiltration. For adrenal glands, this technique is virtually pathognomonic for benign disease when the signal loss is uniform.

Fat saturation

This technique is ideal when an expanded range of soft tissue signal intensities and decreased phase artifact from moving tissues containing fat is desired. Improved demonstration of tissue with a high protein content (e.g., normal pancreas) or detection of subacute blood are important uses for $T1$-weighted fat saturation techniques. When used following administration of gadolinium-based contrast media, the removal of the high signal intensity of fat results in easier discrimination of diseased tissue (e.g., diseased bowel or peritoneum, breast cancer, musculoskeletal neoplasms or inflammation). Fat-suppressed spin echo or spoiled gradient echo imaging is also useful in assessing the fat composition in certain masses such as adrenal myelolipoma, colonic lipoma, or ovarian dermoid cyst. Unlike out-of-phase gradient echo techniques, in which the maximal signal loss occurs in tissues where the fat and water are of equal proportions, fat suppression is maximal when the fat content in the tissue approaches 100%.

STIR

Musculoskeletal imaging benefits from the use of STIR imaging because of the relatively high signal from diseased tissue. Images resemble those obtained using fat-suppressed $T2$-weighted spin echo techniques. STIR is not as sensitive to magnetic field homogeneity as fat saturation and therefore is well suited for imaging small anatomical regions, regions away from the magnet isocenter, or for regions where there are large differences in magnetic susceptibility, such as the cervical spine. STIR sequences acquired using TI times for fat and for silicon suppression are useful for the investigation of breast implant rupture. Because long TR times are necessary, most implementations of STIR incorporate an echo train in order to dramatically shorten acquisition time. Performed as a breath-hold scan, this technique has achieved clinical utility in liver imaging.

17.4.2 *T2-weighted techniques*
Standard multiecho spin echo

Standard multiecho spin echo techniques are used when subtle differences in $T2$ between normal and diseased tissue are expected. A long TR (greater than 2000 ms at 1.0 and 1.5 T) is used to minimize TI saturation of most tissues, though CSF and other fluids are significantly suppressed in signal due to saturation. A short TE (less than 20 ms) is used to produce proton-density-weighted images while a long TE (80 ms or greater) generates $T2$-weighted images. Gradient motion rephasing is normally used on the long TE image in brain and spine imaging to minimize flow artifacts from bright CSF.

Echo train spin echo

ETSE techniques are useful when high spatial resolution or decreased imaging time is desired for $T2$-weighted images (e.g., brain, spine, or pelvic imaging). These sequences are best used when $T2$ differences between normal and diseased tissues are significant since they result in an averaging of $T2$ information. Use of very long TR (greater than 3500 ms) allow coverage of anatomical regions and reduce the amount of signal loss from CSF saturation. Caution should be employed when using ETSE techniques for imaging the liver, particularly in the investigation for hepatocellular carcinoma, because the $T2$ difference between the tumor and background liver may be slight. This is normally not a problem if this technique is used in conjunction with spoiled gradient echo, either 2D or 3D, immediately following administration of gadolinium-based contrast media, as the latter technique is the most effective method for lesion detection.

Fat saturation

Fat-suppressed *T2*-weighted spin echo is useful for liver or musculoskeletal imaging. It results in a decreased phase artifact from respiratory motion of the abdominal wall and provides an expanded dynamic range of tissue signal intensities and increased conspicuity for focal lesions. It is an excellent technique for imaging capsular-based disease (e.g., hepatosplenic candidiasis or metastases spread through peritoneal seeding) since competing high signal from fat is removed and chemical shift artifacts are absent. Fat saturation can also be applied to echo train and single-shot echo train sequences. It is essential to use fat saturation when performing *T2*-weighted ETSE sequences of the liver to attenuate the signal of fat in the setting of fatty liver, because the high signal of fatty liver on nonsuppressed ETSE sequences can mask the presence of liver lesions. The use of fat suppression on *T2*-weighted sequences also facilitates the detection of lymph nodes, which appear relatively bright against a background of low fat signal. For single-shot ETSE sequences incorporating fat suppression, a more uniform suppression is obtained using inversion recovery combined with excitation spoiling.

17.4.3 Sedated or agitated patients

Optimal MR imaging results require cooperation from patients to minimize motion artifacts. For brain, spine, or musculoskeletal imaging, pads or restraints may be used to restrict patient movement. For abdominal imaging, patients who are unable to hold their breath because of sedation or decreased consciousness cannot be imaged with breath-hold imaging. Spin echo sequences may produce images of good quality in sedated patients, but poor image quality may result in agitated patients. Use of reordered phase encoding or navigator echoes may prove advantageous. For dynamic scanning following administration of gadolinium-based contrast media, images can be obtained using slice-selective 180° inversion pulse prepared snapshot gradient echo sequences (e.g., slice selective TurboFLASH, IR-prepared GRASS) followed by either regular or fat-suppressed *T1*-weighted spin echo techniques.

Patients who are unable to hold their breath or who are slightly agitated require imaging using rapid techniques that are motion insensitive. These include snapshot inversion pulse prepared gradient echo sequences for *T1*-weighted images and snapshot ETSE for *T2*-weighted images. These techniques are less sensitive to respiratory motion and acceptable image quality may be obtained. Imaging studies of sedated patients can produce results of good quality when combining breathing-averaged spin echo or navigator echo-based techniques with single-shot approaches.

References and suggested readings

Achten E, Boon P, Van De Kerckhove T, Caemaert J, De Reuek J, Kunnen M (1997) Value of single-voxel proton MR spectroscopy in temporal lobe epilepsy. *AJNR: American Journal of Neuroradiology* **18**: 1131–1139.

ACR (2013) *ACR Manual on Contrast Media: Version* 9.

Bernstein MA, King KF, Zhou XJ (2004) *Handbook of MRI Pulse Sequences*. Elsevier Academic Press, Burlington, MA.

Block T, Frahm J (2005) Spiral imaging: a critical appraisal. *Journal of Magnetic Resonance Imaging* **21**: 657–668.

CKD Work Group (2013) Kidney Disease: Improving Global Outcomes (KDIGO). KDIGO 2012 Clinical Practice Guideline for the Evaluation and Management of Chronic Kidney Disease. *Kidney International* **3** (Suppl.): 1–150.

Debatin JF, McKinnon GC (eds.) (1998) *Ultrafast MRI: Techniques and Applications*. Springer-Verlag, Heidelberg.

De Graaf RA (2007) *In vivo NMR Spectroscopy: Principles and Techniques*, Second edition. John Wiley & Sons, Ltd, Chichester, West Sussex, England.

DeYoe EA, Bandettini P, Neitz J, Miller D, Winans P (1994) Functional magnetic resonance imaging (FMRI) of the human brain. *Journal of Neuroscience Methods* **54**: 171–187.

DIN (2008) *Magnetic Resonance Equipment for Human Application – Classification Criteria for Pulse Sequences*, PAS 1081. Deutsches Institut für Normung e.V.

Dixon WT (1984) Simple proton spectroscopic imaging. *Radiology* **153**: 189–194.

Edelman RR, Wielopolski P, Schmitt F (1994) Echo-planar MR imaging. *Radiology* **192**: 600–612.

Finelli DA, Kaufman B (1993) Varied microcirculation of pituitary adenomas at rapid, dynamic contrast-enhanced MR imaging. *Radiology* **189**: 205–210.

Govindaraju V, Young K, Maudsley AA (2000) Proton NMR chemical shifts and coupling constants for brain metabolites. *NMR in Biomedicine* **13**: 129–153.

Guyton AC, Hall JE (1996) *Textbook of Medical Physiology*, 9th edition. W. B. Saunders, Philadelphia, PA.

Haacke EM, Brown RW, Thompson MR, Venkatesan R (1999) *Magnetic Resonance Imaging: Physical Principles and Sequence Design*. Wiley-Liss, New York.

Hendrick RE (ed.) (2005) *Glossary of MR Terms*, 5th edition. American College of Radiology, Reston, Virginia.

Henkelman RM, Bronskill MJ (1987) Artifacts in magnetic resonance imaging. *Reviews of Magnetic Resonance in Medicine* **2**: 1–126.

Hetherington HP, Pan JW, Chu W-J, Mason GF, Newcomer BR (1997) Biological and clinical MRS at ultra-high field. *NMR in Biomedicine* **10**: 360–371.

Kanal E, Barkovich AJ, Bell C, et al. (2007) ACR Guidance Document for Safe MR Practices: 2007. *American Journal of Roentgenology* **188**: 1447–1474.

MRI Basic Principles and Applications, Fifth Edition.
Brian M. Dale, Mark A. Brown and Richard C. Semelka.
© 2015 John Wiley & Sons, Ltd. Published 2015 by John Wiley & Sons, Ltd.

Kingsley PB (2006) Introduction to diffusion tensor imaging mathematics: Part I. Tensors, rotations, and eigenvectors. *Concepts in Magnetic Resonance* **28A**: 101–122; Part II. Anisotropy, diffusion weighting factors, and gradient encoding schemes. *Concepts in Magnetic Resonance* **28A**: 123–154; Part III. Tensor calculation, noise, simulations, and optimizations. *Concepts in Magnetic Resonance* **28A**, 155–179.

Kuo PH, Kanal E, Abu-Alfa AK, Cowper SE (2007) Gadolinium-based MR contrast agents and nephrogenic systemic fibrosis. *Radiology* **242**: 647–649.

Kvistad KA, Rydland J, Vainio J, Smethurst HB, Lundgren S, Fjøsne HE, Haraldseth O (2000) Breast lesions: evaluation with dynamic contrast-enhanced T1-weighted MR imaging and with T2*-weighted first-pass perfusion MR imaging. *Radiology* August, **216**(2): 545–553.

Le Bihan D (ed.) (1995) *Diffusion and Perfusion Magnetic Resonance Imaging: Applications to Functional MRI*. Raven Press, New York.

MacFall JR, Charles HC, Black RD, et al. (1996) Human lung air spaces: potential for MR imaging with hyperpolarized He-3. *Radiology* **200**: 553–558.

Marks MP, de Crespigny A, Lentz D, Enzmann DR, Albers GW, Moseley ME (1996) Acute and chronic stroke: navigated spin-echo diffusion-weighted MR imaging. *Radiology* **199**: 403–408.

Mezrich R (1995) A perspective on k-space. *Radiology* **195**: 297–315; *Radiology* **199**: 874–785.

Mills I (ed.) (1989) *Quantities, Units, and Symbols in Physical Chemistry*. International Union of Pure and Applied Chemistry, Physical Chemistry Division. Blackwell, Oxford, UK.

Mugler JP, III, Brookeman JR (1988) The optimum data sampling period for maximum signal-to-noise ratio in MR imaging. *Reviews in Magnetic Resonance Imaging* **3**: 1–51.

Mugler JP, III,, Driehuys B, Brookeman JR, et al. (1997) MR imaging and spectroscopy using hyperpolarized ^{129}Xe gas: preliminary human results. *Magnetic Resonance in Medicine* **37**: 809–815.

Mukherji SK (ed.) (1998) *Clinical Applications of MR Spectroscopy*. Wiley-Liss, New York.

Nazarian S, Roguin A, Zviman MM, et al. (2006) Clinical utility and safety of a protocol for noncardiac and cardiac magnetic resonance imaging of patients with permanent pacemakers and implantable-cardioverter defibrillators at 1.5 tesla. *Circulation* **114**: 1277–1284.

Neil JJ (1997) Measurement of water motion (apparent diffusion) in biological systems. *Concepts in Magnetic Resonance* **9**: 385–401.

Nitz WR (1999) MR imaging: acronyms and clinical applications. *European Radiology* **9**: 979–997.

Oosterwijk H (2000) *DICOM Basics*. Cap Gemini Ernst & Young.

Parker DL, Guilberg G (1990) Signal-to-noise efficiency in magnetic resonance imaging. *Medical Physics* **17**: 250–257.

Pinker K, Stadlbauer A, Bogner W, Gruber S, Helbich TH (2012) Molecular imaging of cancer: MR spectroscopy and beyond. *European Journal of Radiology March*, **81**(3): 566–577. doi: 10.1016/j.ejrad.2010.04.028. Epub 2010 Jun 4.

Pipe JG, Chenevert TL (1991 A progressive gradient moment nulling design technique. *Magnetic Resonance in Medicine* **19**: 175–179.

Port M, Idee J-M, Medina C, Robic C, Sabatou M, Corot C. (2008) Efficiency, thermodynamic and kinetic stability of marketed gadolinium chelates and their possible clinical consequences: a critical review. *Biometals* **21**: 469–490.

Prüssmann, KP, Weiger M, Scheidegger MB, Bösiger P (1999) SENSE: sensitivity encoding for fast MRI. *Magnetic Resonance in Medicine* **42**: 952–962.

Runge VM, Nitz WR, Schmeets SH, Schoenberg SO (2007) *Clinical 3T Magnetic Resonance*. Thieme Medical Publishers, New York.

Salibi N, Brown MA (1998.) *Clinical MR Spectroscopy: First Principles*. Wiley-Liss, New York.

Sandstede JJW, Lipke C, Beer M, et al. (2000) Analysis of first-pass and delayed contrast-enhancement patterns of dysfunctional myocardium on MR imaging: use in the prediction of myocardial viability. *AJR* **174**: 1737–1740.

Semelka RC (2005) *Abdominal-Pelvic MRI*, 2nd edition. Wiley-Liss, New York.

Shellock FG (2009) *The Reference Manual for Magnetic Resonance Safety. Implants and Devices 2009.* Biomedical Research Publishing Company, Los Angeles, CA.

Shellock FG, Crues JV (2004) MR procedures: biologic effects, safety, and patient care. *Radiology* **232**: 635–652.

Shellock FG, Spinazzi A (2008) MRI safety pdate 2008: Part 1, MRI contrast agents and nephrogenic systemic fibrosis. *Am J Roentgenol* **191**: 1129–1139; Part 2, Screening patients for MRI. *Am J Roentgenol* **191**: 1140–1149.

Slichter CP (1996) *Principles of Magnetic Resonance*, 3rd edition. Springer-Verlag, Heidelberg.

Sodickson DK, Manning WJ (1997) Simultaneous acquisition of spatial harmonics (SMASH): fast imaging with radiofrequency arrays. *Magnetic Resonance in Medicine* **38**: 591–603.

Sodickson DK., McKenzie CA (2001) A generalized approach to parallel magnetic resonance imaging. *Medical Physics* **28**: 1629–1643.

Sommer T, Naehle CP, Yang A, et al. (2006) Strategy for safe performance of extrathoracic magnetic resonance imaging at 1.5 tesla in the presence of cardiac pacemakers in non-pacemaker-dependent patients: a prospective study with 115 examinations. *Circulation* **114**: 1285–1292.

Stejskal EO, Tanner JE (1965) Spin diffusion measurements: spin echoes in the Presence of a Time-Dependent Field Gradient. *Journal of Chemical Physics* **42**, 288-292.

Tannús A, Garwood M (1997) Adiabatic pulses. *NMR in Biomedicine* **10**: 423–434.

Thomsen HS (2014) *ESUR Guidelines on Contrast Media*, Version 9.0. European Society of Urogenital Radiology.

US Food and Drug Administration. (2006) *Information on Gadolinium-Containing Contrast Agents*. Center for Drug Evaluation and Research. http://www.fda.gov/cder/drug/infopage /gcca/default.htm.

US Government (2008) *Code of Federal Regulations*, Title 21, Volume 8, Subpart B, Section 892.1000, revised 2008: Magnetic resonance diagnostic device (21CFR892.1000).

Vaughan JT, Snyder CJ, DelaBarre LJ, et al. (2009) Whole-body imaging at 7T: preliminary results. *Magnetic Resonance in Medicine* **61**: 244–248.

Wilke NM, Jerosh-Herold M, Zenovich A, and Arthur Stillman A (1999) Magnetic resonance first-pass myocardial perfusion imaging: clinical validation and future applications. *Journal of Magnetic Resonance Imaging* **10**: 676–685.

Wolff SD, Balaban RS (1994) Magnetization transfer imaging: practical aspects and clinical applications. *Radiology* **192**: 593–599.

Wong EC, Buxton RB, Frank LR (1998) A theoretical and experimental comparison of continuous and pulsed arterial spin labeling techniques for quantitative perfusion imaging. *Magnetic Resonance in Medicine* **40**: 348–355.

Young IR (2000) Notes on current safety issues in MRI. *NMR in Biomedicine* **13**: 109–115.

Index

Note: Page numbers with prefix 'f' refers to figures and 't' refers to tables.

atom
  structure of, 2

MRI Basic Principles and Applications, Fifth Edition.
Brian M. Dale, Mark A. Brown and Richard C. Semelka.
© 2015 John Wiley & Sons, Ltd. Published 2015 by John Wiley & Sons, Ltd.

Printed and bound by CPI Group (UK) Ltd, Croydon, CR0 4YY

27/10/2024

14580195-0001